The
Anatomy
of CHANGE

The
Anatomy
of CHANGE

A Way to Move Through Life's Transitions

Richard Strozzi Heckler

Foreword by Robert K. Hall, M.D.

North Atlantic Books
Berkeley, California

Published by
North Atlantic Books
P.O. Box 12327
Berkeley, California 94712

First published in 1984 by Shambala Publications
First North Atlantic Books publication 1993

Cover illustration by Ariana Strozzi Heckler,
   based on a photograph by Jan Watson
Illustrated by Masami Daijogo
Cover design by Paula Morrison
Printed in the United States of America

ISBN 1-55643-147-3

The Anatomy of Change: A Way to Move Through Life's Transitions is sponsored by the Society for the Study of Native Arts and Sciences, a nonprofit educational corporation whose goals are to develop an educational and crosscultural perspective linking various scientific, social, and artistic fields; to nurture a holistic view of arts, sciences, humanities, and healing; and to publish and distribute literature on the relationship of mind, body, and nature.

4   5   6   7   8   9   /   02   01   00   99

To Dr. Randolph Stone, who showed me that compassion and strength are of the same spirit.

And to Maharaj Charan Singh and Chögyam Trungpa, Rinpoche, for teaching me how to sit; Magda Proskauer, who taught me how to breathe; Doris Breyer, who taught me how to stand up; and aikido, for teaching me how to move ahead.

Contents

Foreword

This is a book about wholistic education. It is also about the mind/
body schism in today's crazy world. But it is much more than that. It
examines in simple terms the very roots of aggression and violence
in our global societies, and our failure to learn the law of love. Thus
it is an important book.

The fact that there are buttons that can now be pushed to self-
destruct the world is a clear reflection of the tension and inner
struggle happening in the lives of billions of ordinary people, the
architects of our societies everywhere. That tension is cultural. Culture has always been the product of the individual human organism.
Society is made by individual people who form groups. In addition,
every person is a composite functioning of two simultaneous processes: the mental and the physical. So it seems important, in our
search for both self-knowledge and knowledge about our societies,

to examine the relationship between these two aspects of ourselves, the mental and the physical.

Richard Heckler investigates this relationship and how, although falsely, they often appear perpetually antagonistic to each other. He suggests that the careful examination of how you go about living your life on this planet is a high priority if you're interested in living sanely. It is only by knowing exactly what is true about our own nature that we can come to an understanding of our penchant for harming ourselves and killing each other.

This book examines our cultural tendency to be preoccupied with the thinking, fantasy, or mental functioning and our lack of appreciation for and interest in the subtle rich life of the sensory or body function. The imbalance cuts us off from viewing the world as it truly is. Instead, we each have our own personal fantasy world. We exploit sensation and the body out of greed, in that personal world. We commercialize the body, but we do not acknowledge the body as a source of learning, an ever-present source of information about ourselves. In that way, the more gentle, the softer feelings like love and tenderness go unnoticed.

This seems to be the condition of international politics today. The symptoms of the condition are fear and mistrust on all sides. The cause can be found in our deep mistrust of our own bodies. We have mistrusted that aspect of our lives where love is truly born. Love is a feeling, and we cannot feel it as long as we devalue the body's most subtle messages.

C.G. Jung made testimony to the same observation when he wrote that there are two basic polar forces in the world: the Feminine Principle and the Masculine. His alarm for the world's condition stemmed from our devaluing of the Feminine Principle and the glorification of the Masculine. We tend to place high value on rational thought, achievement, and goal-oriented action at the expense of that part of our experience that is not rational: namely feeling, intuition and emotion. The latter are sensate phenomena. They are qualities that can only be appreciated through the medium of the body, which offers its information via sensation, often in very subtle ways.

In this book, Richard Heckler is writing about the need for balance in our collective psyche and in the physical environment. He points to self-awareness as the tool for attuning ourselves to the world. He is suggesting, in a straightforward way, that we must re-educate ourselves, and that we must change our educational institutions to do so. The change in our orientation to life and education must be a radical one.

His work, and the work of the Lomi School, of which he is co-founder, has been, for the past fifteen years, a systematic exploration of new methods of wholistic education. That work addresses, directly, the need to awaken appreciation for the treasures of information the body offers.

I have had the good fortune to work with Richard Heckler in developing the curriculum and the teaching at Lomi School. For a long time, we have been friends and have shared the same vision. Both the friendship and the vision have never faded. It is a vision of a world where bodily life itself becomes the very ground for mutual respect and caring in human relationships.

This book is Richard Heckler's offering toward the realization of that vision. It is a rich offering, full of wisdom and understanding that can only be acquired from experience and disciplined effort. His excitement and inspiration shine out of his words. Excitement and inspiration are the qualities of a good educator.

Robert K. Hall, M.D.
Lomi School
Mill Valley, California

Preface

"My primary process of perceiving is muscular and visual."   Albert Einstein

I come from the tradition of the bodily arts. As a young boy my early education emerged from the many playgrounds, gyms, basketball courts, and judo classes I discovered in the various places where I grew up. In those environments, I found meaning for my life and respect from my peers. To be a player meant acceptance, fellowship, and an identity as someone who had something to offer. That world also offered the dream of rising out of playgrounds and into the big time. The dream was rarely shared openly, but when we all got together it surfaced from our collective unconscious in the nicknames we gave each other and in the ways we emulated those who had made it. Our games and play held the promise of rising above the average, of doing more than just pumping gas at the local station or ringing up sales at the liquor store.

Later, as I became more involved in the world of organized sports, I learned about working together with teammates toward a common goal. It was in this world of running, jumping, throwing, catching, hitting, risking, and making contact that I also learned what everyone learns in a bodily art: There is a real and important difference between what people say they can do and what they actually do. With this understanding, I took as my teachers those who could embody what they said. I began to learn how to distinguish between those who knew things and could say them, and those who could do those things and be them. I watched how people moved, how they corrected for their mistakes, how they responded in pressure situations. I saw that anyone could talk a good game and that it was easy to criticize from the sidelines, but all that became just chatter when the game started. I began to recognize a certain quality of presence in those who were both concentrated and relaxed with what they were doing. I learned that the reality one made for oneself came from actions and putting words on the line, not from idle boasts. In the martial arts we say, "Put it on the mat," which means to take your philosophy and see what it looks like in action and deed. This continues to be a guiding principle for me, and I feel grateful for having learned it so young.

In the summer before I entered high school, I fractured my knee playing baseball. After the cast was removed, I was encouraged to run and lift weights to strengthen the leg. I continued running and won a track scholarship. I became the first person in my family to go to college. By the time I finished my undergraduate studies, I had been running competitively for over nine years. Among many other things, those years taught me the value of practice and discipline. This was the second important principle I learned from the bodily arts: If we practice and apply ourselves, it is possible to change, grow, and be transformed.

During my years in college, I also experienced a crucial and confusing separation in my life. I moved in two different and separate communities but never felt entirely comfortable in either one. One was the world of the mind and the other, the world of the body. The frustrating distance between these two worlds was, in many ways, what initiated the journey that has brought me to this book.

As an athlete, I delighted in the aliveness I experienced in working with my body. My memories are those of bright sun on my back, the feeling of nervousness before a race, the smell of freshly cut grass during workouts, the heaving breaths that reached to my socks after a hard race, the feeling of satisfaction after exerting myself completely and wholeheartedly. Those experiences added a passion and vividness to my life.

At the same time, I found very little inspiration from the locker-room crowd. I enjoyed the camaraderie, but something was missing. I felt that I was more than just an organized group of muscles training to win a race, and I wanted more. I found some of what I wanted in the intellectual and artistic community. I was inspired to a larger view of the world through literature, poetry, and psychology. But that heady world, with its rarefied atmosphere, often left me stale and with no feeling. I loved the ideas and philosophy, but the lengthy discussions in smoke-filled rooms seemed to have nothing to do with living out beautiful ideas. The two communities were worlds apart, yet there was something for me in both of them. So I went to the physical education building to feel my body and to the classroom to exercise my brain. The distance between the gym and the classroom was the same separation that existed between my mind and body. I was an athlete and I was a poet, but I also felt that I was something more than either one. I felt that if I could discover what the other thing was, the two sides would be united.

In seeking something more, I found that the world of traditional psychology and philosophy did little for me with its arid and complex view. I was also reminded that I learned more from people and actions than from concepts. The spiritual communities that I participated in offered something in the way of a practice and structure to live life by, but they also seemed ungrounded and lacked ways of dealing with emotional and interpersonal issues. Many of the body approaches seemed too mechanical or overly scientific. Most sports and dance looked at the body as a machine to perform on command and then to forget about. Medicine and many body-work systems saw the spirit as simply a higher nerve ending. I was looking for a path that included the bodily life but that also recognized that we are more than our bodies. I wanted a path that worked with the person and the spirit but that also included the body, with its rich array of feelings, sensations, emotions, and energy.

In seeking a form that united these two worlds, I found a workable blend in aikido and the martial arts, the principles of meditation, and a body-centered psychology. These forms revealed to me that our basic life energy, or excitement, is the ground from which the many parts of ourself come to form. I discovered that both my feelings and my thoughts emerged from a limitless current of energy, and that I could participate in shaping them into a total, unified expression. Here there was room for the poet, the scholar, the athlete, and the gambler. The torch bearer and the shadow were birthed from this current and were either restrained or brought to maturity in its rhythms and intensities.

Equally important, if not more so, were the teachers that embodied these forms, men and women who inspired me by their actions and showed me how to use these disciplines. I thank them and continue to thank them for their generosity and patience.

I don't work with the body to exalt it or to conform it to an external image of beauty. I work *through* the body, to discover who we are and how we can cultivate certain qualities in life. In this sense, body refers to the shape of our experience. Everyone is included: the aged who are too feeble to get out of bed, quadriplegics who have no use of their limbs, crawling infants, professional athletes, business executives, housewives. I work through the body for these reasons: (1) our culture has become imbalanced, leaning toward cognitive learning, and has lost touch with the wisdom of the body; (2) the body is a way of accessing people and their deeper urges and potentials; (3) through the body we can learn how to embody the values and qualities we think important; and (4) experiencing the life of the body brings us into contact with the quality of compassion, something that is surely lacking in our troubled world.

I have no particular answers, and I am still discovering and renewing the ideas I have set forth in this book. What I am suggesting is an approach in working with ourselves and others that includes the whole person. I also need to acknowledge the difficulty of writing about something that is basically a nonverbal experience. I've struggled with this on every page of this book, and this struggle has helped me more clearly understand what I do and what I think is important. My hope is that through this struggle I have also communicated with you about the body and the wisdom in *its* language.

Acknowledgments

I would like to thank Wendy Palmer-Heckler for her continual support, inspiration, patience, and generosity during this project. I also want to thank Django and Tiphani for their patience and goodwill during my times of impatience and irritation; Robert Hall for his friendship, generosity, and encouragement; Thomas Pope for feedback; Jacki Fromme for typing and feedback; Robert Nadeau for inspiring many of these ideas; Mutsumi Daijogo for her bodhisattva work with children; Kim Tong for support; Mary Hey for her editorial sword; Emily Hilburn for seeing this manuscript to completion; and the many people I have come into contact with at Lomi School and Tamalpais Aikido dojo.

BACKGROUND

INTRODUCTION

This book is about the journey that returns us to the wisdom of our body. How we can learn from this wisdom to be self-educating and self-healing will be our goals. The first chapter, "The Body of Knowledge," is a plea for a return to the wisdom of the body. It examines how traditional eduation, with its emphasis on conceptual and abstract thought, has denied the potential of the body. The price of this imbalance is reflected in our society as an escalation of crime and violence, a myopic and systematic destruction of the environment, and escalating health problems associated with stress and anxiety. The next chapter, "Working Through the Body," outlines the approach that this book takes when it refers to a return to the body. Working through the body emphasizes contacting our life energy, or élan vital, as a way of coming closer to our deeper urges and potentials. Though many methods may be used in this approach, such as touch, breath exercises, movement, expression, or meditation, our focus is to connect with our unconditioned self, rather than to try to release tension, align our posture, or have an emotional release, although all of that may happen along the way. The chapter called "The Conditioned Tendency" explains how our neurosis can be experienced in the body and how the awareness of this experience is invaluable in helping us move from mechanical, destructive behavior to a more awake and alive way of being. "The Rhythm of Excitement" sheds further light on our bodily felt neurosis, or conditioned tendency, by describing the different ways we squeeze off or overexaggerate our natural energetic cycles. Through case studies, this chapter shows that by contacting our personal bodily rhythm we can establish a working ground to come into harmony with ourselves and with a more universal rhythm. In the chapter "Living in the Body," we learn how to direct our attention inward to awaken the perceptive skills of feeling and sensing. In this awakening we become embodied, which is to say that we experience our life and meaning from the feelings and sensations of our body and not simply from our fantasies and projections. A case study outlines the steps one goes through to live in the body. The chapter that follows, "The Anatomy of Change," describes how the intelligence of our body can be used to help guide us through obstacles and times of crisis. The five stages of moving through change are explained, and practical exercises and illustrations are included. The chapter "Presence and Contact" goes on to explain that by living in our body we can generate a presence that has the power to allow genuine contact with our most inner core, with others, and with the environment. It also describes how energetic presence and contact are the foundations of healing and education. The last chapter, "Taming Aggression: The Aiki Way of Conflict Resolution," accounts for the bodily roots of violence and aggression. In a plea for everyone to take responsibility for their own aggression, by personally experiencing it in the body, this chapter also offers aikido, a modern Japanese martial art, as a way to help resolve the conflict that is so common in our personal and larger world.

In this journey our violence, tenderness, conditioning, and possibilities of a richer and more harmonious life will emerge, but always within the context of being self-educating, self-healing, and self-knowing. My hope is that the ideas and experiments offered in this book will encourage you to pursue the experience of knowing yourself, the world, and those in it. Through my experience, I have come to believe that by living close to our bodily and energetic processes we may lead lives of increasing wholeness and purpose. This book is an invitation to share the principles of that journey.

THE BODY OF KNOWLEDGE

"And what do we teach our children in school? We teach them that two and two makes four and that Paris is the capital of France. When will we teach them what they are? We should say to each of them: You are a marvel. You are unique. . . . You have the capacity for anything. . . . And when you grow up can you then harm another who is, like you, a marvel?" Pablo Casals

We are the thinking animal. Other animals know, but we know we know, and this has become our bread and butter. Through evolution, we have developed a brain that has produced the capacity for logical and rational thinking. These mental skills have rewarded us with tremendous power over the environment and make up the favored paradigm of the pursuit of knowledge. The nurturing of this talent for abstract thought, which has given us such things as tools and medicines, is what is supported by our educational system. We are schooled that knowledge is the result of distancing ourself from what we are to learn. We are told to look at our subject from afar, to dissect it, to put it into manageable compartments, and then to put them into logical order. Instructed to channel our excitement into thoughts, reason, and logic, we have become skilled in manipulating concepts.

There has also been a price to pay for this homage to the power of cognitive mind. Assigning the mind as director of information and learning encourages us to be spectators and not players. We have forgotten the ways of self-healing and self-learning. People of industrialized nations are beset with back problems, high blood pressure, indigestion, headaches, heart ailments, and other ills associated with stress and anxiety. Violence and crime are reaching epidemic proportions, and our addictive milking of the earth for natural resources is myopic. The Cartesian dictum "I think, therefore I am" has left us imbalanced in that we know things but know little about living, about compassion, or about our needs and the needs of those around us.

The majority of us live our life based on what we think and how we order our thoughts. We are keen, educated, and respected individuals who have oriented our life around logic and consecutive thinking. But somewhere along the line our thinking, conceptual world fails in holding our life together. Perhaps we have been unexpectedly left in a relationship, contracted an illness, are unable to effectively express ourself, have fits of uncontrollable violence, or suddenly become anxious and afraid. Yet all of our thinking, ordering, and knowing, makes no difference. Everything seems out of control, and the prevailing view of knowledge, which puts the mind as ultimate authority, is no longer useful or even helpful.

The feelings and sensations that come out of these kinds of situations can no longer be denied or dominated by thoughts. The body begins to have its say, and it demands to be heard. If we refuse to listen, it speaks even louder and we find ourselves sick, numb, or chronically injured. This is the body's way of telling us that we are out of sorts with ourself.

When this happens we need to listen to our body more sincerely and with greater attention. Instead of avoiding or rationalizing our feelings and sensations, we need to hear them as information that can guide and heal us. These points of discomfort are doorways that we can use to begin living in our body. Living in our body means experiencing life through our feelings, sensations, and interactions and not simply from our projections and memories. When we begin to open to and live in our body, whether through pain or joy, a whole new universe of alternatives becomes available to us.

Traditional education encourages us to live society's image and discourages us from awakening to our deeper and more energetic impulses. We learn, but we don't learn *how* we learn. We are not taught how to use ourselves in the learning process. Without knowing that, we lose our individuality by following the images that society and the media systematically place in front of us. We bury the intelligence of our body in order to be uniformly responsive and predictable, which marks the death of preverbal, preliterate wisdom. Disassociating from the wealth of feelings, sensations, images, and intuition that is the inheritance of the body creates a frustration and tension in us. Our contemporary ills and anxieties signal this imbalance. A return to the life of our body would reinstate our heritage of self-education and self-healing. Being responsible for our own health and learning brings us closer to our own source of power.

Somatics, a word derived from the Greek, defines the body as a functional, living whole rather than as a mechanical structure. Somatics does not see a split between the mind and body but views the soma as a unified expression of all that we think, feel, perceive, and express. In the art and science of somatics, we are encouraged to become the source of our information by participating in our knowing and self-discovery. We become the source by contacting our body. In doing so, we bring to light the dimensions of gesture, stance, attitude, emotion, and that which is the foundation of all life: energy (or excitation or excitement). The somatic way of life does not discount thoughts and thinking but integrates them with the *how* of ourself. *How* we actually are, in action, attitude, and the way we relate to others, is the basis for experiential learning. If we embody our ideas and opinions, we can participate more deeply in who we are and who we may become, and we will have at our disposal the primary ingredient for learning: ourself. In whatever situation, the most difficult imaginable, the most delightful, the most boring, we have on twenty-four-hour call what is necessary for making a decision, for taking a risk, for choosing and responding. When we learn how to work with our excitement, there surfaces an aspect of ourself that is rich with information and creativity.

Classroom emphasis on the memorization of facts, formulas, and figures gives us latitude in our social and economic life, but it does little to teach us how we can move through our transitions, or how to work with new and difficult situations. If we begin, however, to pay attention to the textbook of our body, we have access to an entirely new wisdom and language. Through our body we learn *how* to midwife ourselves through the births, maturings, and countless tiny deaths that form the continuity of our life. Connecting with our excitement, which shapes our body, thoughts, and all living things, gives us the possibility of fully living our life. Through our body, we learn *how* to trust and respond to the ocean of excitement that moves us. Living only in our thoughts can make us clear thinkers, but it atrophies our capacity for compassion, intuition, and genuine, felt sharing.

It's not that thinking is necessarily bad. If the world of the intellect is not used as an evasion, the sharing of ideas with others can be a rich and meaningful experience. But when our world of symbols, thoughts, images, and visions is not grounded in lived experience, it tends to become hollow and pretentious. We all know people who can speak with great certainty and righteousness but who cannot live their lives. Often they do not even have a ground or discipline to practice their vision. Their ideas are good, but those ideas have little meaning if they are not embodied.

Living in our thoughts out of a fear of what we may feel and express makes us rigid and unspontaneous people. Out of this fear our mental pattern becomes rigid notions of what it is to be a spiritual person, or what a good parent or leader should be, or how a true artist should live, and on and on. Adopting roles based on ideas that have no ground in lived experience is a distraction from what truly gives us satisfaction and fulfillment. Finding ourself failing to become the symbol that we have adopted, we usually collapse into depression or aggressively defend our symbolic identity, or we blame parents, spouses or institutions for our failures. People with disembodied lives are individuals who, in accepting the societal image, have become orphans to themselves.

I once had dinner with a man who was the president of a prestigious law school and who had been on a number of presidential cabinets. He was an intelligent, informative, and witty man who obviously understood the machinations of power. He sat relaxed and confident, with his head turning this way and that, like a well-oiled turret on his large and unmoving body. His clarity, his depth of vision, and his ability to see the entire range of a topic was impressive. But it was also clear that he had very little sense of his body. He was obviously out of touch with his feelings, and he was the first to admit that emotional experiences had no place in his life or profession. "What does it matter that he has no bodily life?" I asked myself. "He is successful, powerful, influential and well respected. If he is all of these things, even while he is out of contact with his feelings, what is the big deal about body?" Yet some important quality was missing. As we continued to be together, it finally became apparent that he lacked the ability to feel and empathize with another's experience.

Because he couldn't feel himself, he couldn't feel others. If he could separate himself from his body, then he could also separate himself from other people. Without the information from his body, he related to people as facts, figures, and abstractions. He had a powerful mind but was without compassion and feelings. I realized how dangerous it is to remove principles from feelings, especially for a man in his position.

Our schools and institutions encourage this kind of imbalance by asking us to still the natural movement of our excitement and to absorb innumerable bits of information. In this state, information is funneled into us. We become swallowers of history, language, and mathematics but are rarely encouraged to let go of that which is not meaningful or relevant. It is important to learn these subjects, but we also need to be taught *how* to sit so we may better receive; and *how* to appreciate the actual process of writing and drawing; and *how* to participate in the joy of flourish when the name we write is connected to who we are; and *how* to follow the interest generated by our deeper levels of excitement. Our educational system, in elevating the brain to command control, has promoted cognitive knowing to the neglect of our deeper knowings. What our society has called teaching is really indoctrination. True learning, receiving the transmission of experience, happens at a level much deeper than cognition. It is in the experience of the lived body that we have the opportunity to contact and learn from the process of being alive.

Our sports programs and physical education classes have also failed to develop a curriculum of body knowledge. Though our athletes, dancers, and martial artists are involved in bodily endeavors, the emphasis is on performance and not on the creative wisdom that comes from living in our body. Our current programs create people who can excel on the playing fields, but they do not show how skills can be brought into the play of life. The prevailing interest in health and fitness, at its foundations, signifies a genuine urge to come closer to the bodily life.

It still manifests itself, however, as an urge to conform to the cultural idea of beauty and health. It is the health-spa mentality that patronizes the tyranny of thinness. A slim waist may in reality be a sucked in diaphragm that constricts the internal organs. The hardened muscles of the weight lifter may act as shields against feeling and responsiveness. Dietary theory is useful, but it does not tap the information about nourishment that comes from deep inside ourself. Jogging is a response to a need for exercise, but we can run for miles and still be totally out of touch with the messages that our body can give us. The urge toward the bodily life is sincere, but we need to be in touch with what is needed from inside and not simply an external image of how to be. We need to listen to and respond to internal messages before we jog ourselves into fallen arches.

The value placed on going through stress and tension, instead of on learning how to skillfully work with it, is reflected throughout our society. Our companies pay us when we are sick; there is no reward, however, for being healthy and staying on the job. The drug companies are overwhelmingly successful in their production of pills that suppress the symptoms and discomforts of stress-related diseases. Then there is the gym-class mentality of mechanical exercises and games. The physical education building is always on the other side of campus and gives only one-half unit of credit compared to three or four units for academic classes. Students are told to do 100 sit-ups and push-ups and instructed to relax and stand up straight, but they are never told how to do it or what it means for everyday life.

An education that connects us with our body would teach us the difference between what we are experiencing and what we are thinking and fantasizing about. When we are connected with our body, the present moment comes more into focus and we can then begin to make decisions from there. The life that is streaming through our body, with its rich currents of temperatures, pulsations, vibrations, swellings, and congealings, becomes our reference point for choices and responses. When we wonder about a direction to take, or an alternative to assess, we can consult the intelligence that resides in our body. This type of education is revolutionary, in the sense that it gives power to the individual. It fosters a way of being that supports and trusts the energy that moves through all living things.

I know a man who is a doctor, and for the greater part of his adult life he made decisions based on how they would look on his resume. And his resume had to look like society thought it should look—the right schools, the right graduate schools, the right internship, the right fellowship, and the right so on and so forth. Then, because he had a stomach problem that his profession couldn't cure, he went to a body therapist/healer who set him on the road to health. The therapist also suggested that he start a body discipline, which he did. It was a martial art, and through it he began to enjoy a newly discovered strength, suppleness, and movement in his body. He praticed every day, and soon new feelings began to appear in all areas of his life. After a while, he realized that his resume no longer looked as he thought it should look. At first he was confused by this, and then he understood that his resume was different because he was a different person. He was a different person because he was making decisions from someplace inside himself, not based on how they would look on a resume. His confusion didn't last long, because he also realized that his life was much more satisfying now. In fact, he didn't know if his "resume" life ever had been satisfying, because he hadn't felt enough to know. He is still a doctor, and a good one, who is dedicated to helping people. In his words, "I used to think that to have a life I was to do these different things, and then I would be something or a somebody. I suppose it was my idea of what it meant to be a successful doctor. Now I realize that I'm many somebodies, not just a single static person who forever remains the same. That's what my resume fixation was: you know, resumes stay the same. When I began to heal my stomach problems and later took up aikido, I realized I wasn't a resume but a person who can have many different moods and feelings. The things I used to care about—resume, good jobs, having the right car—don't mean as much to me now. I just feel myself differently, and I'm enjoying what I do. So I do my work, which I love, but really I feel like I'm doing my practice all day long. So if something goes out of whack, I don't get thrown off like I used to. I just feel so much more accepting of the hard times, and I enjoy the good times more."

What is missing in our educational system is experiences to acquaint us with our inner knowing. Instruction in the life of the body would establish the conditions for this knowing to take place and for the development of a type of responsibility that would increase our ability for self-healing and self-learning. The goal would be an educational environment where the principles of grounding, energy, centering, expression, balance, contact, relaxation, skillful action, and positive receptivity are learned through the body.

Learning the principles mentioned above would serve two main purposes. First, it would cultivate an appreciation for our basic forms of excitement and expression and of the ways to participate in their fulfillment. Second, it would create a foundation for further learning and for working with the confusion and transitions in our everyday life. This means that whatever form our education might take—computer training, trade apprenticeships, vocational training, study of science or art—learning bodily principles would undergird it. This energetic and bodily foundation would provide the soil from which further learning and growth could take place. Fulfilling these two purposes is what this book is about.

There are a number of techniques that can be used to contact the body and the wisdom it has to offer. We can do deep-tissue body-work for postural alignment; we can use a softer touch with gentle movements for reeducational work; we can use breath and sounds for contacting the emotional character; we can use massage and guided images for relaxation; we can use pressure points, diet, exercises, and acupuncture for health; and we can use conscious movement to develop grace and harmony. But regardless of the method or technique, it is the approach, or attitude, that determines the direction and depth of the work. In the next chapter, we will look at what it means to work *through* the body.

THE APPROACH

WORKING THROUGH THE BODY

"Man has no body distinct from his soul"   William Blake

The intention of this chapter is to clarify the approach this book takes in awakening the wisdom of the body. In light of the multitude of current bodywork methods and the recent fitness boom, it seems absolutely necessary to be clear about what it means to work *through* the body.

We can simplify our understanding by categorizing bodywork approaches into three different groups: working on the body, working with the body, and working through the body. Working on the body is dealing directly with the physical symptoms and ailments that affect our functioning in the world. Included here are systems such as chiropractic manipulations, deep-tissue bodywork, massage, acupuncture, polarity therapy, diet, and proper forms of exercise. They are used to alleviate chronic ailments such as back pain, headaches, constipation, fatigue, muscular tension, and so forth.

Working with the body uses systems such as deep-tissue bodywork, breath work, sounds and expression, movement disciplines, and stress reduction exercises, to enhance emotional freedom and ease of movement.

Working through the body, which is the focus of this book, is contacting the basic life energy that moves through each individual, and the emotional character that is formed from this energy. All of the above techniques may be used in this approach, but the attitude or point of view that exists is fundamentally different. To work through the body is to work with our internal experience and not simply to strive for a better posture, alleviate a physical symptom, elicit a certain emotional response, or be able to move more grace-fully, although all of that may happen.

This approach says that we are our body and that we are also more than our body. In it we are moving toward the most essential part of ourself through the body. Working with the person living in the body, we say "Relax yourself around your jaw" instead of "Relax your jaw." The body becomes a doorway to more refined states of awareness, and through it we can discover the principles of living and creativity. In working through the body, we refer to the body as the shape of our experience—the emotional, intellectual, and spiri-tual shape, as well as the physical one.

To work through the body is not to perfect the body or glorify it. Working through the body is unearthing a wisdom that is often neglected and denied in our society. This is the wisdom of feeling, compassion, and intuition. This way of experiencing knows that a quadriplegic, confined to a wheelchair, can be fully embodied. It also knows that someone without arms can still possess the ability to reach out, to give and to receive, that being grounded is not neces-sarily a function of the legs. To be a grounded person is a function and expression of the spirit, of our attention and energy and how they move through the body. At its most profound, the goal of work-ing through the body is to allow the universal spirit or energy, that which unites and is the source of all life, to guide and inform our lives.

To work with someone through their body is to be interested in the qualities, capacity, and rhythm of their energy. To see the person through their body is to see how they contain their energy, how they express it, and the ways they awaken it. The way we relate to our energy system is also the way we make contact, and the way we make contact tells us what brings meaning to our life. Our many levels of energy and how energy moves through the body tell us who we are in the present and what we have denied in the past. How we rigidify who we are, and how we seek that which we long for, can be seen in the way our energy interacts with the world.

Working through the body, we contact the person and their energy in the way they gesture and move, the sound of their voice, their urge toward or away from contact, their posture, how they respond under pressure, and how their images and thoughts are translated into action. The way we feel, think, express, and interact, in other words, reflects our energetic rhythms. To work through the body is to first perceive patterns of excitement and the energetic rhythm of expression rather than the cognitive organization of specific issues. To work energetically is to work with the context of our life and not only the content. The way someone is, in other words, tells us much more about them than what they say or profess.

To work through the body is to contact the person at three levels: the present situation, or "what is" about them; the past, or the historical patterns that shaped them into the "what is" of their present reality; and the future, or what now wants to come to life as expression and vitality (usually what has been repressed in the past).

The first step in working through the body is to bring attention to "what is" in our experience. This part of our energy is most in the foreground, and it determines how we are most likely to respond when in a stressful situation. It is the energetic expression that has been most useful for our emotional, mental, and physical survival. By looking at "what is" in ourselves, we can see how we have embodied our attitude toward life. For example, if we are listless, vague, and without motivation, that will be revealed in the tone of our musculature and in the ways we quiet and dim our energy, or in such things as the flatness of our voice or our inability to breathe deeply. Whatever the case, we must first bring awareness to "what is," and not to necessarily change it. We can do this by amplifying our energetic quality through movement, touch, or sound or by simply being quiet and experiencing it deep within ourself.

Once we have contacted "what is" about our situation, the history of how we have become this way may emerge. It can surface in feelings, memories, or images of the past, and they may provide insight into the present situation. This history can be present in the body as contractions, rigidities, distortions, or chronic squeezing. By working through the body, these emotional wounds can be revealed and integrated into who we now are. But working with the past is important only if it is not a diversion from what is presently being lived. Working through the body is to return again and again to the energy that is being experienced and lived in the present moment.

The third step is to see what wants to come to life, which may be an urge to change jobs, or a growing desire to let go of an old anger, or perhaps an unexpressed need to finally accept happiness and love or a reaching out for contact. Some part wants to move forward, to evolve into a new way of being, to find a new way of expression and a new quality of excitement.

Whatever the urge, in this step the way to work is to interrupt the old conditioned way of responding. This evokes a startle response, which creates an opening and a fresh sense of aliveness. In the opening, we can introduce exercises, forms, and practices that bring life to the part that has shriveled and grown dim and that encourages that which has been denied and is now seeking expression. These exercises work with attitudes, muscular contractions and expansions, gestures, breath, and internal states of being. They are designed to contact the person through the body and not to be used as mechanical procedures that program a certain set response.

Regardless of the situation—whether we have an excessive aggressiveness that pushes people away, a grasping that frightens others, a criticalness that is cold and aloof, or a seductiveness that manipulates others—to work through the body is to encourage us to go beyond our need to understand the whys of ourself and into the actual experience of who we have become bodily. It is embodiment that brings us to the experience of being responsible, mature people who are capable of making decisions and living the values we hold to be important.

To now begin the journey into our bodies, we must first know, through experience, when we are not living in our body. By contacting the physical setting of our neurosis—our conditioned tendency—we gain the ability to recognize how we disconnect from ourself when confused and in transition. This recognition is the necessary beginning in moving toward embodiment and using ourself as our source of learning. By simply looking at what is, we are able to feel how we shape our body, thoughts, and language in a way that removes us from the present situation. Experiencing our conditioned tendency creates a ground from which we can begin to live in our body.

THE GROUND

THE CONDITIONED TENDENCY

"Mr. Dufy lived a short distance from his body."   James Joyce

In the course of our development we make certain choices, consciously and unconsciously, to insure our physical, social, and emotional survival. These kinds of choices create attitudes that, in turn, shape our experience of the world. If the situation in which a choice is made is traumatic enough, an attitude can be formed in a single crucial moment. Other times, an attitude forms over time in response to a certain consistent communication. The choices that lead to the forming of attitudes involve some sort of compromise, so what we do is sacrifice some part of ourself in order to survive. It is like crippling or stunting part of ourself so that the whole may continue. In some sense, this self-wounding is an intelligent act in that it is necessary for survival; at the same time, it also becomes the core of our neurosis.

Here's a simple but contemporary example. A young child, after being with the babysitter for the day, sees his mother coming down the street. As he excitedly runs toward her, a neighbor fires up his gas-driven lawn mower. The child could respond in many ways at this point, but let's say he is frightened, and his joy at seeing his mother turns to fear as he runs to her crying. After picking him up, the mother quickly says, "It's okay. There's nothing to be afraid of now." But the child is still genuinely afraid, and he continues crying. She demands that he stop and says that if he doesn't she will put him down. Thinking that he may be separated from the object of his love, his terror increases and he cries louder. She puts him down. In order to be reunited with his mother, he tightens his jaw and holds his breath to numb his fear and inhibit his crying. The mother then picks him up and confirms his response, saying, "That's a good boy."

If this episode is crucial enough, or if it is repeated regularly, the child will learn to deal with his fear, terror, or perhaps any unexpected change by holding his breath and compressing his jaws. The message is that if you want approval and love, get over your tears and fear quickly. And the message creates an attitude, that to be weak and vulnerable is not acceptable. This attitude, which is commonly held, is muscular, has a physical location, and affects the way we relate to life. In our example, the young child will carry his attitude in the way he clenches his jaw and constricts his diaphragm. If the attitude sets in, that is, if he can no longer relax his musculature and express his feelings, then it is not uncommon for other symptoms to appear. Ear, eye, teeth, and headache problems may occur because of the clamping jaw, or asthma, lower-back pain, and indigestion may arise from holding in the diaphragm. The emotional consequences of these rigidities may be expressed as sudden and violent rages in an otherwise quiet, "good boy" type of person.

We all have our conditioned ways of responding. When our state of balance is upset, our system is flooded with a stream of energy. Thrust into a potpourri of thoughts, feelings, and sensations, we become disoriented and confused. Illness, breaking off a relationship, taking a new job, deciding to move, arguing with the boss, or learning a new skill can all put us in transition.

In an effort to restore familiar ground during a crisis, we check out of the situation as it is, ignoring the energy that is streaming through us, and adopt a known, conditioned way of behaving. This is the *conditioned tendency* which is, in effect, the physical setting of our neurosis. Some of us become defensive; others of us shrink and become small. We may intellectualize the situation and never feel it. We all have a personal wall that we construct to separate us from any reality that we disagree with or that throws us off balance. It is a way of being, an identity we can assume when we feel that on some level our survival is threatened. This tendency, as I mentioned earlier, is shaped by some event or events, usually in the context of our family, the schools we attended, our religious training, or the neighborhoods we grew up in—in brief, the environments of our social and moral upbringing. At some point in our development, our conditioned tendency was valuable and useful for our survival. The present question is, "Is it now useful and relevant?"

When our conditioned tendency emerges, our muscles set in a particular way. We assume a specific posture, breathe a certain way, take a stance, literally, that manifests the tendency. This tendency, which is actually imprinted in the flesh by many years of practice and use, takes over, and in some critical way we lose touch with the present moment. It is as if we become unwilling to open to the tremendous amount of energy that is released when our status quo is upset.

Working somatically offers us the opportunity to physically and energetically experience how we *become* our conditioned tendency, that is, how we become identified with our conditioned tendency. Because it is literally in the flesh, blood, and bone of things that we act out our changes, it is natural to use the body as a way to pay attention to ourselves as we expand, contract, and move through our lives. Simply, the physical form is the place where we live out our lives. Using our body, we can feel how our excitement moves through us when we are aroused; we can perceive our uptightness when our shoulders begin creeping up to our ears. Paying attention to our breath, we can learn about our emotional state. Our conditioned tendency, the style in which we relate to the world, is naturally related to the life of our body.

Our conditioned tendency can take many forms, but intellectualization is by far the most common form of diversion and evasion. Cognitive knowing is often a way to circumvent feeling. Becoming overinvolved in our thoughts is a way to avoid the emotions, gestures, and expressions that were at some time in the past responded to unfavorably or with disapproval. In order to emotionally survive disapproval, we rationalize our dilemma. Cutting off our natural urges and excitement, we alter ourselves into an acceptable form to become good boys and girls. While we are thinking about how to please, our guts are a raging fire. Conditioned to act according to the wishes of others, we squeeze off part of ourselves; we find ourselves left with lifeless arms that were scolded not to reach out, constricted throats that were told not to speak too loudly, pelvises pulled back from sexuality.

Other people rebel and do everything they can to defy their oppression. These are the people who have shaped themselves into an unrelenting No! These are the perennial adolescents who are still fighting battles that should have been fought years before, while they were happening. When this is our stance, we even struggle with those who wish to serve our best interests. We automatically lock into a fighting posture and lose the ability to discriminate. We become unable to receive what is nourishing or to discard what is irrelevant. When the unexpected occurs, we will usually respond defensively. We will tend to think that we are being taken advantage of and then construct a defense. We may tense our legs and feet to hold ground, for example, and not release the breath fully, creating a false sense of size and strength. Yet, because we lose flexibility, this muscular and cognitive attitude actually weakens stability and creates more vulnerability.

Whatever choice we make, timid and acquiescent, puffed up and defensive, or aloof and distant, the subsequent emotional surgery divides us into many parts and gives us anxiety about who we are. We siphon part of ourself off to make sure we don't rock the boat. Always looking over our shoulder lest we make the wrong move, we find it difficult to organize ourself into a unified, self-forming expression.

But it is in the conditioned tendency, the neurotic shaping of ourself, that we can also find the ground for working with our imbalance. This shaping is the manure that enriches the field of who we may become, the context to bring forth that which we have long withheld. Constricting the diaphragm, for example, to limit sensations of longing in the chest requires a great deal of energy. But if we exaggerate the constriction, or use breath, movement, and touch to release it, or simply allow our attention to be with the experience, we are working directly with the energy of that conditioned tendency. This same energy, whether it is used to contract or to expand, can provide the ground for becoming more of who we are. This way of using ourself is very different from simply talking about how we got to be the way we are and trying to make logical sense of our predicament. We may have interesting insights, but if we also work with the excitement itself, the enactment of our life can become richer and more fully alive. Blending insight and embodiment is having a vision while our feet are planted firmly on the ground. The way we walk on this ground then becomes our journey and path toward the vision.

Gerard

Gerard began to work on himself during a transition in his life. As a corporate executive, he had enjoyed success in his professional life but had been unable to maintain any kind of ongoing intimate relationship. His relationships with women always ended with their leaving him, and he felt considerable bitterness about being rejected. After years of faulting the women for leaving, he was beginning to consider that it might be he, or at least partially he, who was playing a part in this scenario of the unfulfilled personal relationship.

There was a flatness, a one-dimensionality, about Gerard that was reflected in his body. There was little tone or definition in his tissues. His movements were determined, cool, and slow moving— glacierlike. His voice had the tone you hear on airport paging systems. But what was most apparent was the lack of movement in his chest. It was as if there were a giant hand pushing forward on his sternum. This caused his shoulders to round forward and his head to droop over the valley of his chest.

Gerard had some vague psychological notion that his mother had something to do with his failure with women. He felt if he could "know" this, and he desperately wanted to, he would discover and solve the core of his problem. He was sure that once he analyzed this business with his mother he would be able to develop a long-term relationship. Though Gerard moved slowly, like a reptile coming toward the sun, his mind moved restlessly, without ever settling in any one place.

I had Gerard lie on his back and experience his breath. I placed my hand on his chest and asked him to experience the contact between us. I encouraged him to stretch and exercise his eyes, so he could see what was in the room instead of his ideas and plans. It was extremely difficult for Gerard to tolerate any sustained breathing in his chest or to surrender to the warmth of my hand on his tissues. In fact, Gerard had difficulty tolerating any increased sensation or feeling. After a few moments of touch or breath, he would break into a violent coughing fit. Gerard was unable to tolerate his own sensations and excitement, yet he still wanted to "know." He would interrupt his breath, his coughing, his feeling, and his visceral life with wanting to know. Knowing was a god at whose altar Gerard sacrificed his élan vital. His neurosis was physically located in his chest, and his conditioned tendency was to defer to his head and to engage in blame when he felt too much. With this information as a working ground, it seemed that Gerard already knew enough.

As Gerard worked on himself, he began to relate more directly with the feeling of compression in his chest, with his fits of coughing, and with the images, symbols, and memories that arose. He initially resisted by continually asking why he would choke on his deep inhalations and by incessantly formulating fantasies that placed him in the company of desirable women. But as he continued to experience his conditioned tendency, he began to open to the life of his body and to discover some remarkable things about himself.

He experienced for the first time the hole and numbness in his chest. This became a point of departure for his realization that he was terrified of intimacy. He saw that when anyone came too close— physically, emotionally, or psychically—he would withdraw by squeezing his throat, chest, and pelvis. Tying himself off this way cut off his ability to make contact and to contain and express his excitement in a meaningful way. He was like a balloon that had been tied off into three separate, noncommunicating compartments. He was unable to form himself into a single unified expression. To release the pressure of his compartmentalized life, he would cough his excitement away, keep his breathing very still, or go into fantasy. He realized that this pattern of tying himself off existed in his social relationships with women and even in his relationships with his business colleagues. As Gerard began to make friends with his conditioned tendency, his willingness to work with himself increased. He didn't feel such a need to skip over his anxiety. He was more open to experiencing his conditioned tendency as workable and not something to make an end run around.

Working with his experience of choking had surfaced the memory of a near drowning he had had as a young boy. This insight was exciting for Gerard, and he wanted to stop and elaborate on it. I appreciated the insight but continued to encourage him to contact the excitement that was tied into the cough. As he moved deeper into his waves of excitement, a sudden rage overtook him, and his voice, suddenly free of coughing and stammering, took a new full-throated dimension. Later he explained that what emerged from the memory of his near drowning was his mother standing by helplessly, afraid to come near him. He reexperienced his outrage over this and how he could never completely trust her again. It became clear that he had unconsciously transferred this mistrust to all women. In his continuing work, he included this valuable insight into restoring life to his imprisoned body.

Gerard's work illustrates that the conditioned tendency does not have to be seen as something that is wrong with us or as a complex problem to solve. Our conditioned tendency can stand in the way of our full capacity, but it can also provide the excitement, the momentum, for moving toward a more satisfying experience of ourself.

Here is a simple example to better illustrate the conditioned tendency. Actually, it is an exercise from aikido where the idea of pressure becomes a living experience in handling various strikes, grabs, and kicks.

In this exercise a partner firmly and unexpectedly grabs your arm, usually from behind. The grab sets off a rush of energy, and the reaction is usually the conditioned tendency. In a group situation, different characters graphically emerge. The shrinker becomes small and disappears under the intensity of the energy; the defender puffs up and prepares for an attack; the intellectual removes themself and studies the situation; the activist becomes busy, scurrying around and adding chaos to an already chaotic environment.

We identify with the conditioned tendency if we are unable to tolerate, or lack experience in tolerating, an intensification of energy. As mentioned before, the response to a sudden or new burst of energy is to check out, that is, to respond inappropriately in a fixed, unconscious manner. What almost everyone reports at the point of the grab is the experience of their excitement moving up, very quickly, into their head. After we are "grabbed" our system is flooded with energy, sensations, feelings, temperatures, movement, vibrations, and pulsations. Unable to tolerate this much life in the moment, we rush to our head, label the excitement that is so overwhelming, and then assume our conditioned posture, which corresponds to the conceptual label. If our conditioning, for example, is to feel guilty about our energy, then we may round our shoulders and lower our head when we are "grabbed." When things get out of control, we try to manage the situation by going to our brains, by "knowing." This trying to restore order with a conceptual label is manifested in a corresponding muscular attitude. The conditioned tendency is an effort to freeze what's going on, and the effort required to do this is uncomfortable, if not painful.

If we don't buy into our conditioned tendency, we have the opportunity to feel the rush of energy as a possible resource in times of change and crisis. Instead of freaking out over the huge rush we are getting from the grab, we can begin to see that this flood of energy may actually be made friends with and that it can provide intelligible information on how to handle the change. We could even say that the energy rush has surfaced to help us deal with the situation.

In presenting this grabbing exercise to a wide range of people over the past years, two distinct insights have emerged. First, it is clear that the person learning a martial art must necessarily first learn how to deal with their own energy before they can properly execute any self-defense techniques. If we do not relate appropriately to our own excitement while under stress, it is unlikely that we will be able to handle an attacker. If we are insensitive to our conditioned tendency, the ways we block and immobilize our own rush of energy, it's a mistake to think that we will be able to manage someone else's energy. Because of this, we first teach people to be settled and familiar with their own excitement before getting involved in technique. In this way, the technique grows out of a feeling of being in harmony with ourself and not the mechanical application of rehearsed moves.

Second, our reaction to this physical grab is the same reaction we have to other forms of pressure, mental, emotional, or interpersonal. It's not as if we have a whole repertoire of tricks and reactions, but rather we have a single response that we have developed and refined. In this sense, the exercise also operates in a metaphorical context. The grab can represent many different levels of experience: the grab of a loved one dying, the grab of paranoia, the grab of someone cutting in front of you in a line. So this grab can be an actual event with an actual energetic response (someone literally grabbing you), and, at the same time, it can tell us who we are in the world, in our daily life situations. It can bring to light in a bodily sense the way we connect with and withdraw from ourself, others, and the environment. It's a research experiment with ourself as the laboratory. Throughout the book, I will refer back to this grab and its metaphorical meaning.

In either context, the literal or the metaphorical, what comes to the foreground is the possibility of seeing the ways we work with and against ourself. The conditioned tendency, or neurosis, is exposed, and, at the same time, it becomes the ground from which we can work toward some degree of wakefulness. This bodily felt neurosis becomes the point of contrast that is so vital in the process of learning and embodiment. By becoming aware of our somatic processes we can actually feel how we set our body into our well-rehearsed tendency: how we lose contact with our feet, lock our pelvis, jump out angrily at the grabber (which could be the boss, our spouse, employees), or contract and become victims of our own energy. Whatever reaction we've majored in, it will emerge as a kinesthetic mood—a bodily experience of the patterns of our energetic nature.

Once we have recognized our conditioned tendency, we can expand this insight by experiencing ourself as being involved in a bodily and energetic process, which is the rhythm of excitement. This rhythm is the basic energetic process that touches all of us in each moment of our lives. To experience this rhythm is the next step in moving toward living in our body.

THE RHYTHM OF EXCITEMENT

"By my actions . . . teach my mind."   William Shakespeare

We all have a particular energetic rhythm or style. We can see it in the way we make contact, the way we move through transitions, how we work or play, the way we bring something into form, or even how we live our days. The first and most obvious thing about our style is that we have an initial tendency to be either extending out or gathering in. Some people are like the antennae of a snail and recoil quickly if they are touched too suddenly. Others are like big shaggy dogs that yearn to be tousled and rubbed with care and affection. The initial response to either move toward the action or collect oneself back in is the same regardless of the situation. It may only be a split second, but it will be there. This is our conditioned tendency. From this initial moving either out or in, we ideally then move into our rhythm of excitement.

Our excitement, in its rhythmic pulse, passes through four distinct stages: awakening, increasing, containing, and completing.

These stages can be used as a map to look at the way we use ourself energetically. This map is not a novel idea; in fact, nature is probably the original author. The stages are much like the cycle of the moon, the rhythms of the tide, a complete breath, or even the structure of a good novel. In the case of the body, our excitement revolves through the seasons of a birth or beginning awakening stage, a period of growing and building, a maturation or containment, and then expression and completion.

Because of our conditioned tendency, which was birthed somewhere in our past and now shapes the way we respond to certain experiences, our rhythm of excitement will inevitably be out of balance. Somewhere in our development we have all had to starve some part of ourself in order that another part might grow and thrive. This makes us stronger in some areas and weaker in others. If we have been taught to fear our intensity, for example, we may never allow ourself to fully express ourself. If we were told to always be positive and expressive, we may be bubbly, "up" people but without the maturity that comes from the containing of our energy. Those of us who learned to be adept at containing may be timid in expression and sharing. Those of us who are always discharging may never allow our energy to mature and ripen. Some of us can start projects but cannot follow through. If crying is taboo, we may learn well how to contain but at the sacrifice of vulnerability and release.

The point is, whether we like it or not, we all have places of balance and imbalance, strength and weakness, neurosis and health. But by being aware of our personal energy style, we are less likely to be caught in traps with ourself. This awareness can broaden and deepen the way we live and also help us form more meaningful relationships with ourself and others.

Our imbalance will manifest itself both in our personality and in our body, and we can use it as an ally in locating our attention and energy. By locating ourself, we can work with our situation instead of being caught in a mechanical reaction. The point is not to try to change our imbalance but to bring awareness to it and to use it as a pivot in working with ourself.

Imagine, for example, that you are the type that starts many new projects but then runs out of gas before things are completed. If you know this about yourself, and I mean know in the attitude and shape of your body, then you will know where to locate your energy when you want to free yourself from your conditioned tendency. People who are good starters will have numerous ideas about beginning new projects, curiosity about many different things, inspirational visions, and quick little bursts of excitement throughout the day. At the same time, they will infrequently follow through on their inspiration. To work bodily with these kinds of issues is to bring our insights into the feeling dimension, in other words, to experience what this imbalance feels like in the body. We focus on not just knowing it but on moving a step deeper and experiencing it in the body and energy field. When we do this, it is possible to mobilize our energy and attention out of our neurosis much more quickly.

Another value in recognizing our particular style is learning that the creative process, which is tied into this energetic rhythm, has its own timing. The reason so many of us are burned-out after a good first novel, record album, painting, or performance is that we do not honor the natural rhythm of the creative process. As soon as we produce something of quality, we are encouraged (and often commanded) to immediately do it again. It is as if we think that the creative process and our excitement can be bottled and mass-produced. But once we start to push ourself inordinately out of our bodily rhythm, our efforts become dull and uninspired. We need to see that although the creative process can be worked with, we have to honor its rhythm and pulse. The first stage in this rhythm is the awakening of our excitement.

Awakening

Most of the people who come to the *dojo* (Japanese for "training hall") for the first time are stunned by the activity, the energy, and the directness of contact between people. Most of these new students are effective and successful in their lives, but in this new situation their familiar world has been replaced by something intriguing but really quite foreign, and maybe even a little menacing. What they do is what most of us do in a new situation: they try hard to do the right thing. This leaves them stiff and about five feet from their bodies. They look like they are under some kind of spell and suddenly cannot tell their right foot from their left. They are simply not present, and it hinders their learning and communication.

What is missing is curiosity. Their intention to perform everything right is sincere, but it does little to bring them into the experience of what is actually going on. What they need to do is to restore their natural curiosity and inquisitiveness by asking, "What do I feel?" or "Am I afraid? Am I excited? Can I see the other bodies moving around me?" These seem like elementary questions, and they are. But if we respond to these questions from our bodily experience, we suddenly come into focus. We may feel the energy streaming in our legs, a tingling in our hands, or the way we control or release our breath. It is this simple curiosity and interest so crucial to the learning process that is missing for most of us when we are in transition or learning something new. Curiosity and interest are key elements in awakening ourselves.

If we have lost our curiosity, our learning is slower, more arduous, and filled with painful memories of past failures. But if we are curious about what we are doing and how we are doing it, our struggle to perform correctly gives way to an inquiry of our hearts, eyes, ears, and feelings. If we follow our curiosity, we become involved in awakening and inspiring ourself.

When we awaken ourself energetically, we are responding to our impulses, desires, and urges. Just as the infant's first knowledge of gravity awakens a process of excitement and discovery, we begin to experience our excitement in response to a desire or urge. The world touches us and moves us through an upset, a transition in relationship or profession, the weather, a meaningful insight, the meeting of a new person. If we do not respond to these urges but simply listen and watch them, we may become quiet and insightful but we do not evolve and expand. Response to desire is the cornerstone of growth. Desire in this sense refers to the deep and ancient impulses that move us toward the more of who we are, not the hankerings after sweets and gratification.

There is a time to quiet ourself so that we may look at and listen to who we are. There is also a time, and a need, to go with our desires and urges. This is the path of passion. It is the making of a seasoned and rich soup that we call our process, the all of who we are.

Curiosity and interest are the key and ignition of our energy; together they have the capacity to turn us on. They do not create new energy but rather allow us to contact the ever-present life energy by turning our attention toward it. When we pay attention to ourself, we can experience a warmth, a movement, a life that arouses us. Desire swells and forms into an intention, blood surges, the adrenal glands begin to expand and release, our tissues vibrate with excitement, and we begin to make contact with the world. When we are not curious or interested, we do not feel our aliveness. This is also true of institutions and organizations. When we, as the

institutional or community body, are no longer curious and interested, rigidity takes the place of aliveness.

Whenever we sincerely ask ourselves, "What's out there? How
am I? Where does this road lead? What is this?", and then allow ourselves to respond to those questions, we ignite our energy and generate ourselves. When this happens there is a pool of warmth that
stirs within us, desiring to grow and be cultivated. The image of our
reptilian ancestors lifting their heads toward the sun and shore as
they emerged from the sea comes to mind. Awakening ourself inspires contact and adaptation, the twin instruments of human evolution.

Asking our children to sit and memorize facts that have no rele-
vancy in their lives dulls their spirits. It conceals the joy that can
come from learning and self-discovery. If we cannot find ways to
bring the spark of awakening to students, and then teach them how
they can generate that spark, we are failing to educate them. If our
educational methods primarily involve quieting excitement, we will
produce quiet and obedient students. These students will become
citizens who will follow orders, who will fight the authorities' wars
and enforce their rules. When we follow blindly, we forget that we
are capable of being curious and interested in life, our own life, and
the lives of those around us.

Jacob

Jacob, who is thirty-three, slouches in his chair. His posture is the
picture of a defeated person. His head hangs far forward of his
torso. It is as if there is a large yoke around his neck that supports a
weight that hangs somewhere around his genitals. The muscles in
his neck and upper shoulders have become taut cables in order to
support this yoke and its accompanying weight. He breathes in a
shallow, uninspired way, and his voice emerges sounding like a
crushed styrofoam cup. Jacob expresses himself through complaints,
and in many ways he has a right to do so. He has suffered much in
his life as he does now. The problem with his complaining is that it
doesn't do any good, and it has become habitual, leaving him without friends or companions. In his burdened, squeezed body, complaining is the only thing that Jacob can do with any consistency. His
main complaint is that he can't get anything going, "I can't get anything off the ground," he says. He can't get anything off the ground
because he's not on the ground in the first place. The colossal weight

that he carries around his neck makes it difficult for him to lift up or begin anything.

Jacob talks about these perceptions and is momentarily thrilled by the mental connections that he makes. But his reasons and motives for what he does seem, like himself, heavy and lifeless. His strategy is to keep putting the ball in my court. He wants me to initiate, to generate the aliveness, to begin something. Weighed down, he has little ability to awaken himself. From his state of self-imprisonment, he looks out at the world, complaining but expecting. Jacob has made himself a loser without an avenue to win; he cannot find his starter button.

I touch Jacob's chest where it is most sunken and ask him what he feels there. After a moment, he says it feels "like a gray, barren plain." When I ask for a feeling and not an image, he collects his attention and spend some time with himself in the area of his chest. After a bit he looks up with a kind of wonderment in his eyes and says increduously, "There is no feeling there." I ask him to say "I feel nothing here" as he touches his chest. His curiosity is aroused, and it presents itself as a focusing of attention. A quality of feeling emerges, and he says, "This deadness feels solid and unmoving." Something is aroused in Jacob, and he becomes involved in a new level of energy.

Because changing or interrupting a set pattern will often awaken our excitement (change any part of your daily routine—don't drink the usual afternoon coffee, take a different route home, comb your hair with your left hand—and see what happens). Jacob, in another session, experiments with a new way of standing. His initial and most practiced form of resistance is to reply that it won't do any good, although he doesn't know what will do any good. I ask him to break the old practiced pattern with something new. He stands with his back about two feet from the wall and bends back with his hands over his head, palms touching the wall, fingers down. He stretches his head back and down and sees how far he can walk down the wall with his hands. It is not far, but far enough to stretch his neck and chest into a new shape. Choking noises sputter from him and huge breaths rush into his neglected lungs. His respiratory and circulatory system experience a new life. His shoulders, chest, and neck are momentarily open in new ways. When he resumes standing, more of his chest and stomach face the world. For a moment he no longer leads with just his head. He stands straighter, with more balance and strength, but also with more vulnerability.

There are new sensations, new feelings. In some way Jacob has taken the first step in beginning a new life. He has initiated a new form; he has ignited his own excitement.

Rachael

Rachael is an illustration of another way of awakening. Rachael's was an energetic awakening through uncovering the origin of her pattern of self-deadening. Through an insight, she generated herself energetically and on the spot.

Rachael felt the need to work on herself because she had lost all of her curiosity and interest in life. Though she was in her thirties and rightfully a woman, she always seemed like a girl. She was frail, sunken in appearance, and drained of any expression. She said that she used to take dance classes, but her muscle tone appeared inadequate to do anything more than hold her up. She had little motivation, and she complained that life was a constant effort. Dragging herself into my office, she would sit forlornly and offer little more than downcast eyes and heavy sighs. Looking at her I would think, "Where is her life? What is she doing with her excitement? How does she manage her life in such a state?"

After a few sessions, interesting things began to emerge that helped draw a picture of Rachael's condition and her inability to awaken her own excitement. First of all, her present state of deadness had begun when she broke up with her boyfriend about six months previously. It was the first time since she was seventeen that she didn't have a boyfriend or a husband. She had always counted on these men to initiate the excitement or motivation to do something. As long as someone else led the way, she could follow. But after her latest separation, she had decided to make a go of it without a man and had fallen into this depression. She was totally out of touch with any impulse or desire that could be carried into action. Rachael had a great deal of courage to face this part of herself, but she was slowly being pulled into a dark, lonely hole.

Rachael was so out of touch with her energy that sometimes it seemed like a great effort for her to even breathe or talk. But remembering an incident that happened early in her life provided the fire for her to move forward.

As a child she was raised without a father, and her mother was away working most of the time. She remembered a time when she was almost seven and being taken care of by a woman whom she feared and mistrusted. As this memory began to surface in Rachael, her eyes began to widen and there was a mounting edge in her voice. "I was outside, and I was trying to learn how to ride a bicycle with a neighbor girl. I remember that we were in some kind of competition about who could ride the bicycle first. At first it was very exciting and fun. We would fall off and laugh and try to make the other person laugh so they would fall off. Then for some reason we became very serious. I don't know why, but all of a sudden there was a lot of tension and pressure, and while my friend began to get better and better, I kept falling more. I tried to start playing again, but my friend became even more serious and soon she was riding her bike. I felt horrible. The defeat and humiliation were overwhelming. I lost, and she taunted me about how she had won and how I had lost."

Rachael stopped in her story at this point. She was looking at something a long ways away, and her breathing began to deepen. She seemed to swell and straighten with each deepening wave of her in-breath. "I felt too ashamed to stay with my friend," she continued, "and there was no one I could go to for consolation, especially not the babysitter." Rachael suddenly sat up at this point with wide eyes and said, "I went to my room and I remember saying to myself, 'What's the use of trying? I won't succeed anyway.' From that moment on I think I lost my will to make any effort to try for something. I told myself that it was not worth it to try and compete because I would never be good enough to win or good enough to enter the competition, so I might as well stay in my room."

When Rachael finished her story, she was quiet for a few minutes, and then her eyes grew big and a smile began to spread across her face. She sat straight up as if someone were suddenly blowing her up with air. "I gave up then," she said. "I went to my room and gave up. That room became me, and I have never really come out." Rachael truly looked like a different person as she spoke. She looked alive. She was making contact. The excitement around this uncovering touched her because it awakened her curiosity and interest.

Rachael worked intensely on herself for a year after this powerful awakening. Although it was very revealing, there was a lot of work to do to integrate this memory and bring it into her present life. At first she wanted to use the experience as a way to pity herself, which threw her back into her inertia and pattern of deadness. Anger then surfaced, but she quickly wanted to repress it because she

didn't know whom she was angry at. The anger kept returning however, and she finally allowed it to surface.

My work was to support her interest and curiosity in whatever
impulse, sensation, or emotion that came to the surface. The initial
work focused not so much on anything specific as on the quality of
her interest and how she responded to her impulses and urges. In
this way, she became interested in following her excitement, no matter how small or insignificant. Bodywork and movement work awakened those parts of her that had gone dead. She would stamp, sing,
throw insults, pound, sweat, and respond in quiet meditative ways to
her deeper yearnings and wishes. Rachael showed that if we stay
with our insights we can bring ourself into a state of aliveness. In
bringing her bodily process and intellect together, Rachael awakened
herself in a way that was previously unknown to her.

Increasing

All of us know people who are constantly inspired but who seem to
have little or no ability to follow through. They are like novas who
have a moment of brilliance and then fade away. You often hear
them saying, "I'm starting to . . . ," or "I'm on the verge of . . . ," or
"Soon I'll begin to. . . ." They always have a great idea or a fantastic
insight, but it lacks the increasing of excitement and tension that is
necessary for an idea to emerge into form. There is no building of
energy into form. Here we have the man who has premature ejacu-
lations, or the woman who goes from man to man, or those of us
who start thousands of projects but never finish them. When we are
caught in this short-circuited pattern of unfulfillment, we become
frustrated and end up blaming others for our lack of success.

Our ability to build on what we have awakened, to continue to
intensify our contact, depends on how we create boundaries for our
excitement. This means that after our initial awakening, we need
to stay with and appreciate the streamings, rushes, and vibrations
that flow through us.

If we have a difficult time with pleasure, success, or satisfaction,
we may have a tendency to abort what we have begun. But if we
decide to stay with and participate in what we have begun, we increase our state of aliveness. If we are unable to tolerate the increasing of our excitement, we also will have little tolerance for others

and their excitement. If we sabotage ourselves because we cannot stand the increased feeling, we will most likely sabotage others when they feel more of themselves.

As we increase our initial awakening, we enlarge and expand our excitement and increase our ability to tolerate deeper levels of contact. Allowing our excitement to build and grow, without being crushed by it or being constantly under its shadow, is to appreciate and work with the intelligence of our energetic life. By attending to our sensations moment by moment, we can build boundaries for our excitement. People who lack the ability to form boundaries to contain their energy are often given to hysteria. When they do not build on the initial surge of excitement, it comes crashing through, knocking them and other people over. If there is nothing between the arousal of our energy and the expression of it, we are swept away in a flash flood of emotion.

It is possible to experience the increasing and forming of energetic boundaries through the flexing and releasing of muscle groups. We can allow a surge of energy to grow into maturity by gently squeezing part of ourself and then releasing. At first, the time given to flexing and releasing is equal. Then, as we are able to contain more, we can reduce the flexing time and increase the releasing time. In a sense, this is a conscious cooling of the first heated eruption and acts just as cooling hot lava, which forms clear boundaries and begins to run in distinct rivers and streams.

In increasing ourselves, we have to remember that we don't necessarily have to do anything with the energy except to stay with it. We need only to be present with ourself by attending to our sensations. Just because we are hit with a jolt of energy doesn't necessarily mean we have a green light for some kind of action. We need to practice appreciating the currents of energy in our cells and muscle fibers without doing anything other than staying with and feeling their power and movement.

Try this. Sit in front of your favorite food or drink. Let's say it's a late afternoon candy bar. Sit down, unwrap it, and put it in front of you, but don't eat it. Experience the urge to eat it, the intention to reach out for it, the desire that moves through you. But instead of acting on these impulses, stay with all of the emotions and sensations that are happening inside you and around you.

Allow the energy that surfaces from the wait to enhance your already awakened state. Let the energy increase by consciously attending to it instead of reacting to it. This is a staying power that is enhancing, a practice in experiencing energy itself. It is making friends with your energy system.

When we plant a seed of awareness and then assist its growth by attending and cultivating it, we are involved in a process of building and growth. If we constantly dig the seed up and see if it is growing, we hinder its growth. At the same time, if we ignore it and don't water it with our attention, it will wither and die. Once we plant the seed of awakening, we need to nurture it in a way that is neither suffocating nor abandoning. If we work with the rhythm of the seed itself, it will blossom in its appropriate season.

Robin

Robin is a painter, and she came to work on herself because she was in an artistic vacuum. After a number of successful shows, she felt unable to follow through with any of her inspirations. She began painting after painting only to abandon them. She was dedicated to her work and felt committed to her artistic journey, yet she found herself hopelessly mired in take-offs that got nowhere.

Robin is a short, intense woman with bright shining eyes. Her life has been filled with travel and many rich experiences, and she has done most of it alone. She said she would like to have a relationship, but she seemed too set in her ways as a single person to really make this happen. Her range of expression ran on a narrow spectrum from sitting silently and motionless to constant fidgeting and uninterrupted monologue. She tended to be overly intellectual and her feet and leg complaints seemed to be a signal for her to pay more attention to the ground and the bottom of her body. Robin lived with her shoulders high around her ears, and for a painter she had very little life in her hands and arms. Her limbs looked like the dangling appendages of a puppet. In talking to Robin, what was most noticeable was that she seemed either so still one wondered if she was present, or so animated that she was discharging all over the room. This made for a prickly kind of contact, as she darted in for short, antagonistic stabs and then quickly retreated.

Robin's portfolio showed the work of an artist who was disciplined, refined, and had a sophisticated aesthetic. Her art was impressive, and so was the difference between her artistic range, which was wide, and her emotional range, which was narrow. Narrow was the word to describe Robin and her rhythm of excitement. She

moved quickly from awakening to completion, without anything in
between. This made it almost impossible to find any space or rhythm
in her contact. She had very little tolerance for building and containing her energy. Her work focused on increasing her energy
within a workable boundary. An increased tolerance for her energy
would widen Robin's ability for contact, and it would strengthen her
creative process.

After a period of getting to know Robin and watching her process of painting, I asked her to lie down and breathe. Her breath
was small and confined to her lower abdomen. Her pattern was to
take a series of small, quick breaths that she occasionally punctuated
with a deeper breath. This deeper breath was almost like a sigh,
which she never quite allowed to mature but quickly blew away.
Robin didn't want to take too much in, and what she did allow in she
held onto very tightly. This gave a panting quality to her breath.

I asked her to image a ping-pong ball at her lips and to allow
her breath to come in and out in a way that would blow this imagi-
nary ball always to the same height. As she began to find a fuller
rhythm in her breath, her energy began to escalate. After a minute
or two of this, she started fidgeting and then talking about something
that was a thousand miles down the road. This returned her breath
to the small rapid panting in her belly. When asked about her sudden talking when her breathing became more rhythmic and full, she
replied, "I feel these tinglings in my body, and they make me feel
very uncomfortable, almost claustrophobic. Then I just start talking.
I don't even know what makes me start, I was just talking. But when
I was talking, I didn't feel the tinglings and I wasn't so uncomfortable."

Robin revealed how the sensations in her body frightened her,
how she thought they would overtake her and that she might be
suffocated by them. Her escape, or release valve was to start talking
and discharging in some way, or she would evacuate to some secret
place deep inside herself. Robin knew little about creating a boundary structure to allow her awakened excitement to grow into some
sense of containment. She had an either/or approach to life. She
needed to be either in total expression or not present at all. But because this expression had no building and containing, it also had no
depth. Robin does have depth, and she is a reflective person. But
because she didn't allow this depth to ripen and mature, she came
across as an idle, senseless chatterer. Since people manage their en-

ergy in the same way regardless of the situation, Robin must have had the same problem in her painting. Her zeal for painting lacked a proper channel to grow into form.

In the next session, I rested my hand on Robin's chest and she immediately withdrew her attention. As soon as she felt sensations building from the touch, she disappeared. It was as if there were a corpse under my hand, where a few minutes ago there had been a person. For many weeks Robin worked with this theme of either departing when she increased her feeling, or becoming expressive almost to the point of hysteria. This was done through touch, through her breath, and with leg and arm movements. The work evolved to a point where instead of going into one of her lengthy monologues for expression, she was able to express this with her body. She learned to kick, pound, gesture, and shout for expression instead of just verbally rattling on.

Once when she was thrashing around on the mat after a series of deep inhalations, I instinctively began to restrain her movements. Robin responded by struggling even more vigorously for a moment, and then she suddenly became very quiet and very still in her narrow sort of way. She must have remained that way for about five minutes. When she opened her eyes, she looked at me more directly and with more sustained contact than she ever had before. I let go of her arms, but she continued to lie there, looking around the room like a young child.

"Let me tell you what happened," she finally said, slowly sitting up, her eyes full of feeling. "I went back to a place when I was very young. I don't know how young, but young. I was in a crib. I had these sores on my body, and my mother was strapping me down so I wouldn't scratch them. I was terrified. I was terrified then, and I was terrified just now. I felt like my body was crawling with insects, and I couldn't scratch them or pull them off of me. It was like being devoured, and I was utterly helpless. I couldn't do anything, and my mother left the room." Tears started rolling down Robin's cheeks and blood began to color her face where previously there had been only a waxy deadness. "My mother had told me about this, but I had never experienced it in such depth. I felt like I was right back there, and it connected to the way I can withdraw my attention. Since fighting against the straps was so useless, I just slipped through some tiny, tiny hole in myself and hid in there until they undid the straps."

This was a huge breakthrough for Robin, and she continued to

have important insights. She also began to have more tolerance for
the building and increasing of her excitement. This happened especially in her contact with close friends.

The next step was to get Robin on her feet, so we went to the
dojo to work with movement. At the dojo, Robin learned a simple
aikido wristlock that, if applied correctly, will bring a person down.
The intention was not to show her a self-defense technique, but to
give her a tool to help her learn how to participate in the increasing
of her energy. So, in this way, the technique became a metaphor.
The initial grab represented her awakening into an inspiration that
wanted to be painted. The continuing pressure, or the wristlock,
represented how she responded to her excitement building toward
the creative expression.

After a few preliminary instructions, I applied the technique to
her wrist, and she began to space out. Her attention floated to the
other side of the room, and her body began to shift away from the
pressure. She became aware of this, and we then did the technique
again. More present now, she immediately screamed that it was too
painful and began to struggle. In the ensuing discussion, she said
she felt claustrophobic. "There was no space," she said, "I felt overwhelmed. This is similar to what happens in my painting."

In the continuing work she discovered that if she didn't inhibit
or slow the energy down, she became unfeeling and her attention
drifted away. She simply became unavailable. Or she would struggle
and fight, which only confined her creativity and movement. In this
way, Robin again saw how she stopped the increasing of her excitement by either spacing out or struggling with the energy itself. After
inspiring herself, in other words, she felt oppressed by the awakened energy and it quickly swamped her like a canoe taking too
much water. Her reaction was fight or flight.

As we continued, I asked her to stay with the sensations in her
wrist, slow herself down, and allow the feeling to empower her as it
intensified. This required a certain inhibiting of the reactions of
panic and spacing out. She began to allow the sensation in the wrist
to enliven the rest of her, to allow a thickening and increasing in her
other hand, in her legs, and feet, in the feelings in her belly. As she
trusted this process, she reported a sense of thickening in herself.
The vibrations and pulsations increased, and she began to feel a
pulse through her torso and pelvis. Robin talked about this experience in terms of sensuality and satisfaction. "It is the same feeling
I have when I'm 'on' in my painting," she reported. "I'm with myself,

but I'm also responding to an inner rhythm. Because I feel good with myself, I feel good about what I'm painting."

After she did the wristlock exercise a few times, we created a new metaphor for her to experience this sense of energetic increasing. In this metaphor, the space off the mat represented the everyday, routine Robin. Stepping on the mat (a distinct feeling difference, especially without shoes) represented her beginning a new painting. The mat became the metaphor for her painting canvas. When she stepped on the mat, she again reacted in one of her two ways: She either took her attention quickly away from the initial experience or she hastily expressed herself without allowing the feeling to mature. This was her conditioned pattern. When she stepped on the mat the third time, she experimented with attending to her experience, slowing herself down, and allowing the thickening to take over. As her energy increased, her knees began to bend slightly, her center of gravity dropped and she reported an overall feeling of tingling and aliveness, and her boundaries felt extended about a foot from her skin. "I feel like I have substance and presence," she later wrote. "This is a pleasurable feeling, almost erotic."

After some work with this process, and dovetailing it with her psychological patterns of resistance, Robin later found it possible to take this metaphorical and literal exercise and adapt it to her painting. She now knows her reactions to increased feeling and how to take an alternative route in tolerating her sensations. This allows her creative process to unfold in concert with the rhythm of her excitement.

Containment

Where I live there is a flood plain where the tide makes its rounds in and out of the bay. When the sea rushes into these wide basins, pressing critically close to the edge of the banks, it seems as if it will overflow into a new tributary. Then the current will suddenly quiet, and the water will find its own level. The tide is no longer coming in, and there is nothing spilling out. A richness of weight and fullness begins to swell out of this holding. The gentle slopes of the basin shape this part of the sea into an alive and pulsating form. Contained into manageable boundaries there is a power and magnetism in the now full marsh. Gulls and ducks form flotillas in the inlets, while cranes and sandpipers step carefully through the reeds in search of food. Sometimes a fish will splash or people will tromp through the marsh grass or gaze idly into the thick, wet belly of water. Soon the tide will flow out, and this body of water will deliver itself into the bay. But there will be a moment, endlessly repeated in this cycle of coming and going, where there will be a containment of fullness and potential.

Containment is a time when our forward thrust into growth and expansion begins to balance off. No longer at the forward edge of seeking and increasing, our energy matures by widening and filling out its boundaries. Perhaps it is in our personal growth, our profession, in a relationship, or in a certain craft that we have this feeling of maturity about who we are and what we are doing. It is a place where we can genuinely say, "I know how to do this, and I find satisfaction in doing it." The increasing of our excitement gives way to a stabilization. We can enjoy the fruits of our efforts. It is pleasurable and fulfilling to feel our boundaries contain us. The push is off and there is a feeling of acceptance about who we are. If the awakening and increasing of our energy is like the upward momentum of a plant, then our fullness is the outward growth of the leaf.

The words maturity, boundary, and containment are meant to convey a sense of ripening and satisfaction, of fulfilling a potential. But if we think of these terms in adolescent standards of curfew and restriction, we resist genuine containment by always being on the move. Never settling into our experience, we never know who we are. Without containment meaningful contact becomes elusive, and our endeavors never ripen into accomplishment and fulfillment.

People who have problems with containment are usually well practiced at awakening, increasing, and completing their energy. They move in the fast lane of life and can accelerate very quickly on the surface of things. Yet if they slow down, they begin to fidget, squirm, and evade. Constantly discharging, they never take root in their experience. Their lives lack depth and a sense of filling out. Like water striders, they skim over the surface of a deep, rich pool.

Initially, these people have the attitude that containing is something undesirable. They say they want to be free spirits, unhindered by any boundaries. Commitment and responsibility are seen as burdens to their springy outlook on life. Underneath this they are afraid of what they will see if they stop and settle with themselves in a sustained way. Beneath the veneer of brightness and drive is a deep insecurity about who they are. They have serious doubts about their capacity to manage the intensity of their energy or to tolerate its vividness. They fear they may become stagnant and uncreative. They wonder if they will be embarrassed by the limits they find in themselves. They are afraid of the shadow they constantly hold at bay.

These people need to work with their staying power. They need to slow down and be where they are. They need to explore how they can tolerate the intense energy that comes with feeling relaxed *and* powerful. They need to practice forms that allow their weight to settle and their spirit to rise. They need to remind themselves to enjoy and relish their fullness. Stop for a while and appreciate where you are. If you can only play one scale on your instrument, stay with it for a while. Contain and develop that experience instead of always hurrying on to the next thing. You will know what you can comfortably contain and when it is time to move on.

Michael's story, which follows, illustrates some of what we have been discussing about containment.

Michael

Michael is forty-one, an executive at a major oil company, father of three healthy children, and has been happily married to the same woman for eighteen years. He has an incredible amount of energy, and he seems to find time for his many activities and the various people he contacts. He is respected by his family, profession, and community. Michael basically likes himself, and he enjoys life. He contacted me because he wanted to work on his golf game.

Because of his position in the oil corporation, Michael was invited to play in a pro-am celebrity golf tournament. Being a competitive person, he wanted to improve his game for this prestigious tournament and thought that feedback through movement analysis and energy work might help.

When Michael was in town, we would meet in a room large enough for him to swing a golf club, or we would go out on the golf course. He is a short, round man with taut spindly legs and a firm protruding belly. If you looked only at his belly you might think him fat, but the all of him didn't give that impression. He was compact, robust, and he never seemed to stop. Even when he was standing still he seemed to be in motion. A low rumbling constantly emanated from him, and his ruddy complexion lit into a fierce brightness.

Like a confident but hungry falcon, Michael was always on the alert for new game. He never seemed to settle anyplace for very long. He was always darting here, inquiring of this, needing to make a call, or flying off to the next destination in an unending rhythm of starting, building, and discharging. There was an omnivorous quality about him as he quickly swallowed food, things, and people, and then moved on. In many ways he was exciting to be around, but being around him all of the time could also be wearing. His constant inventory of observations, opinions, insights, and pronouncements were both very entertaining and, in the long haul, exhausting.

As Michael worked on his golf game, this scenario of constant motion began to surface. He hurried himself and it showed in his game. He lacked the particular sense of balance and power that comes from settling into something and taking time with it. The lack of this missing piece that we are calling containment was evident in many areas of his life. Whether at play or business or with his family, Michael kept himself from any sustained contact. Never allowing his energy to establish its natural balancing point, Michael always kept on the go.

Early on it was clear that it was important to focus on this imbalance in Michael instead of rearranging his golf technique. If he worked with the quality of energy that is associated with containing and deepening, his technique would naturally and automatically begin to adjust. He was always churning, and that set the stage for just about everything he did. In his golf game this appeared in two specific ways. First, he couldn't hit the long ball with any regularity and he had an almost zero average with long putts. Always being in flight, Michael's center of gravity was never low enough to acquire the needed balance and strength that was necessary to hit with power or to putt with sureness and confidence. Second, he couldn't pace himself well when he had to play more than eighteen holes in a day. Because he was unfamiliar with an effortless stride, he would prematurely wear himself out. Once Michael made an offhand remark that pretty much summarized this part of him. He said, "I enjoy starting things and getting them rolling. Then I like to hand the job to somebody else so I can go on to the next project."

Michael's curiosity became aroused as he saw his pattern emerging. He began to put a number of things together, and our work started to overlap between counseling, bodywork, stage presence, sports, and therapy. He explored this new dimension in his life from a place of inspiration and interest. He didn't doubt what he had accomplished or who he was; he simply and genuinely had an urge to know himself. . . . and to improve his golf game.

There were a number of ways that Michael worked on his pattern. Sometimes he would focus directly on the elements of his golf game. At other times we would work directly with his muscles and tissues. Working deeply in his connective tissue or moving his limbs in supportive ways taught him how to use the appropriate effort for an action. Sometimes he would lie down and work with the capacities and qualities of his breath. He also learned certain energy states in the aikido dojo, and throughout the work we would discuss and exchange ideas.

There is a basic strategy in working with someone in a specific discipline (golf in this case, but it could be dance, tennis, acting, martial arts, drawing, marksmanship). The first step is to recognize what is, and then to see what is missing, what is out of balance. Then one must interrupt the old pattern. This evokes a startle response, which in turn creates an opening and excitement to work with. Then the person is given new forms and exercises to practice and use in the newly opened space.

In Michael's case, what was missing was the containing and empowering of his energy. What made his life out of balance was his compulsive running from one thing to another. Though his golf game was the primary reference point, he was open enough to look at his patterns in other areas of his life and interested enough to go deeper. One of the most fundamental and startling things he saw was that his low level of tolerance for pleasure and satisfaction was at the heart of his avoidance of containment. He simply wouldn't allow himself to settle into his accomplishments long enough to gather the fruits of meaning and satisfaction. He remembered his mother driving into him the importance of getting ahead, staying on the move, and being innovative and dynamic. He was full of stories and impressions that equated busyness with effectiveness. What was apparent to everyone but Michael was that he was a naturally innovative and dynamic individual. His staying-in-flight syndrome only got in the way of it.

Once Michael had a dream that reflected his imbalance. "I am walking through the rain, head forward, shoulders hunched like a fullback fighting for a first down," he said. "I seem to be walking for miles like this when suddenly I stop, straighten up, and let my shoulders relax. It is as if I realize that I don't have to fight the rain and that there is noplace I really need to get to. With my head up, I notice the rain has stopped and everything around me is bright and sunny. I stop by a small lake and quietly lie on the grass." Later he remarked, "I see this dream as that part of me that struggles with life and never stops to see the beauty around me. It's the fullback in me, who considers gaining yardage as the purpose of living."

After he told this dream, we began to interrupt his pattern of skating exuberantly but superficially on the surface of life. Right before the beginning of his golf swing, for example, I would have him wait. When he would hurry after his ball, I would encourage him to slow down and find a natural stride in his walk. He began to take time with the approach to his shot instead of just stepping up to the tee and firing one off. At first this frustrated him, but it also initiated new levels of alertness and excitement. Breaking his pattern opened the possibility of choice and new ways of experiencing.

He also experimented with his breath pattern, which was high and dominated by the out-breath. He would lie down and breathe in his belly and enjoy the feeling of expanding on the in-breath. He also began a sitting practice, sitting forty minutes a day. In this time he learned to simply observe his intention and desire to move, without responding to it. Whenever the urge arose to get moving, which it did often and with surprising aggressiveness, he would practice using the energy of that reaction to settle and deepen in himself. In his breathing pattern his instructions were to allow the in-breath to mature and ripen, and not to exhale so quickly.

Walking on the golf course, he would experience what it was to have a pace or stride that is effortless and effective. He worked with his center of gravity and legs in his putting and long drives. Soon he began to enjoy the experience of his legs being rooted. He felt a new and unexpected potency in his thighs and feet as he deepened into them. He always knew they could run; now he was discovering they could anchor him and draw sap from the earth, nourishing him and investing him with power.

Breaking up Michael's old pattern of constant escalation carved out a space for him to practice new forms to acquaint him with the experience of containment and deepening. He was introduced to something that had been a stranger to him, and he made friends with it. What he needed was to feel forms, actions, emotion, and muscular attitudes that expressed this state of containment. Michael genuinely began to change, from the way he walked, to how he related to his children, to his golf game. On all fronts, Michael began to operate from a more contained place in himself.

Michael did improve his golf game, but more important, he also felt that he was given an alternative. A choice was uncovered that gave him an added sense of freedom and aliveness. He could now appreciate and participate in a level of contact that was unhurried and fulfilling.

Not that Michael no longer moves through the world in constant motion. This is an integral and exciting part of Michael. He finds meaning in this way of being in the world; it makes him successful at work, and he is, of course, both loved and resented for it. But that would be the case in any event.

Completion

In *kyudo*, the Japanese art of bowmanship, the moment of releasing the arrow is called *hanari*, or the loose. It is a result of *kai*, or union. It is an incredible moment where the fully drawn bow, in synchronization with the mind and body of the archer, can no longer contain the energy of the union position, and the arrow is spontaneously released. *Hanari*, in other words, grows naturally out of *kai*. As a famous *kyudo* master said, "When the time is ripe, the arrow flies, as a fruit falls from a tree." To see a master archer at the moment of *hanari* is a breathtaking view of beauty, timing, and effortlessness. There is no sense of shooting the arrow at a target. The arrow flies simply because it is what must occur next. It is a poetic completion of dignity and daring.

This is a particularly appropriate image for the stage of completion in the rhythm of excitement. What it conveys is that completion is a natural extension of the stage of containment, not a product of a mental decision. Our gyrations about completions and endings— "Should I go now?" "Have I done enough?" "Can I stop now?"— come from the separation we place between ourself and what we feel. The creative satisfaction that comes from completing something emerges from our energetic experience and not from what we think. Think of the full bladder that naturally wants to relieve itself, the out-breath that emerges from the full expansion of the lungs, the iris of the eyes that closes when it can no longer tolerate more light, the natural fall into sleep that ends the day. Completing the energy of contact, like *hanari*, involves the creative and spontaneous discharge of energy. Just as the release of the arrow makes room for the next one to be notched, completing a particular cycle of contact ends what has come to form and also makes space for a new beginning. When we learn to make closures and end chapters, we can then freely move ahead to challenge new boundaries. Many people who have come to some kind of ending in their life find themselves at a loss as to how to manage it. Out of touch with their rhythm of excitation, they usually react in one of three ways: they cut short something that is not yet ended, they cover over the ending with inappropriate affection, or they try to keep life in something that is truly finished.

Those of us who tend to evacuate a situation prematurely will often do so by creating an unpleasant situation. After a time of closeness and shared intimacy, we predictably start an argument when it begins to end. We will start to blame, fade away, or begin something new before completing what is at hand. If we are able to provoke others into being angry, we have created a self-fulfilling prophecy and can say, "Your anger tells me that our intimacy doesn't mean anything, so I will leave." When this happens there is a shadow that is cast over the affection and care that has been shared. Some part of us wants this, of course, as it justifies our fear of contact and intimacy.

There are others of us who avoid endings by quickly reaching out to hug or fill the situation with inappropriate affection. This is more seductive and often more compelling than the first strategy, but it is still a way of avoiding a deeper and more complete ending. Such affection or hugging is respectable escape. Not wanting to feel the pain of separating, we shield ourselves with a syrupy kind of contact that denies any possibility of a genuine completion.

Then there are those of us who linger and hold on even after the contact is clearly over. A form has completed its cycle, but we go to great efforts to keep it alive. We become tired in our life because we expend energy keeping a relationship, a job, or some endeavor afloat when it actually started sinking years ago. Many of us, for example, cling to the anger and resentment we have toward our parents as a way of avoiding the responsibility of adulthood. As long as we hang on, we can continue to blame others for our lack of fulfillment. Endings are a natural part of the rhythm of excitement, and without them nothing new can come to form. If we leave things prematurely to avoid saying good-bye, or if we hang on for the same reason, our beginnings are crowded with the ghosts of the past.

If we are fearful of our emotional life, or have been taught strict taboos about expressing certain feelings, we may not be able to completely end something. But by inhibiting our emotions during a time of endings, we carry these feelings into our life. This casts us into a shadowy world somewhere between the living and the dead. If anger, for example, is forbidden in our self-image, then the anger that was appropriate but unexpressed at a particular ending will find its way into some part of us. As a burning spark it will smolder in our muscles, organs, and attitudes, finally making us sick. Then this repressed anger from the past inappropriately boils over in other situations: we become angry at our children, our employees, the boss, ourself.

When our lives are filled with, in the words of Fritz Perls, "unfinished business," our body may begin to signal these incompletenesses in a number of ways. If someone complains that they have been recently troubled by headaches, constipation, cramps, blurred vision, lower-back pain, what have you, they need to ask, "What am I leaving uncompleted? What am I holding on to? What is my body telling me to complete more fully?"

Working with our completions, we see if our storyline matches our energetic experience. If someone says they are relieved that a relationship is over, and at the same time they are grinding their teeth, they need to focus on the energy of the locked, tense jaw. If someone says they want to continue with a relationship, but their body says there is no longer satisfation in it, they need to listen and respond to the messages and needs of their body.

There are no prescriptions or formulas for dealing with endings and completions other than listening to the energy of our body. To say endings should be managed in this way or that ignores the richness and complexity of our life. In completions that are guided by our energy, we are able to say, "This form no longer holds my excitement," or "I no longer have energy for this level of containment," or "What was once nourishing and informing no longer excites or interests me."

Tom

During his early twenties, Tom turned toward meditation as a way to work with a tremendous grief and suffering in his life. The particular meditation practice he chose was one that emphasized watching the different emotions, thoughts, feelings, and sensations that arose out of his sitting meditation. The practice and teachings of this path had a powerful effect on him, and they helped steer him through his difficult times. This practice developed his concentration, his ability to have an objective witness to his experience, and the insight of the impermanence of phenomena. His practice helped him become less hysterical and fragmented. He learned how to contain his excitement and find workable boundaries for his experience. He liked what was happening to him, so he began to relate to the world through the framework of his meditation.

Years passed, and at some point he began to use containment as a wall to separate himself from others and his own experience. His practice began to rigidify into an ideology that rejected some experiences and favored others. Certain emotions, like anger, were bad. Others, like joy or delight, were seen as simply not useful. His contact with others became limited to watching them, just as he watched himself. If things got a bit rocky he would immediately, as an evasionary tactic, take his attention to his breath. He was concentrated and contained, but the rest of him was numb. After a while, he began to lose touch with what he felt, what his values were, and how he made decisions. He could watch, but he couldn't respond. Behind his front of serenity and confidence, he was scared as hell. Friends left him because of his arrogance and lack of feeling.

Working with Tom was in one respect quite easy. He understood how to use his attention, and he was willing to look at himself and to work with what he saw. But he was also difficult to work with because he was so much in control. He was always carefully holding himself together. He had developed the quality of containment into a solitary, watchful tower that stood sentinel over everything he did. He had an awareness of his body—the sensations, temperatures, the rising and falling of the breath—but he didn't know how to be his body, to be informed by it, to live in it. Excitement would arise and he would contain it. Feelings and emotions would begin to surface, and he would put them in a holding pattern. "It's important to stay on center," he would say. If he suddenly erupted into a spontaneous gesture, it would embarrass him. Tom gave the impression of giving, but he never gave of himself. He gave objective information like theory, facts, and philosophy without ever revealing himself.

Tom went slowly in his work. We built a solid foundation of trust that allowed him to slowly come out from behind his emotional stockade. He loosened the large muscles in his shoulders and legs so he could kick, stamp, swing, and reach out. He softened the areas around his eyes and jaw so tears and laughter could flow easily from his taut face. He learned that he could follow his excitement instead of just watching it. After a time, he came to the grief that initially brought him to his path of meditation. Because he now had the tools for containment, he felt less frightened about going into his feelings of grief, rage, and mourning. He began to soften, and out came many emotions, feelings, movements. He would allow his containment to complete into expressions of feeling or self-knowing. In one session, a fury broke loose from him that was both terrible and wonderful. He was a volcano, and when he was through erupting he said, "The world seems so much closer to me now. I don't feel like I have to defend against you or anyone else. I have been so busy watching and holding myself, I forgot about living. I see now that I was always saving myself, but I didn't know for what. It feels so nourishing to freely spend myself."

Tom still meditates, and he has become somewhat of a leader in his spiritual community. When you meet him it is still the reserve and containment that initially stands out. But he also has a twinkle in his eye, and he laughs more freely at himself. People now say that they trust him more because he lets them know when he is angry and because he is more open with his opinions and judgments. He is more willing to let go of his reserved contained space and express himself.

Having established a working ground through the experience of our conditioned tendency and the four stages of our rhythm of excitement, we can now turn toward what it means to live in our body. In the following chapter, we will see that to live in our body we must feel and be aware of the sensations, temperatures, streamings, weight, and pulsations of the body. When we become embodied in this way, we are in a position to draw from the intuition, power, and insights that the body has to offer.

THE WAY

LIVING IN THE BODY

"He who feels it, knows it more."   Bob Marley

I once was hired by a juvenile detention center for adolescent males
to consult as an aikido teacher. On the first day a kid who was about
six-foot-three charged at me when the group was released into the
exercise room. I moved quickly out of the way, and he said to me,
"I'm so pissed I could kill someone." He was already a criminal of-
fender, and I believed him. I turned to him and without really
thinking said, "Well, I'll show you how to kill somebody, it's easy."
This stopped him for a moment, but not knowing whether to believe
me or not, he just kept up his hard-ass macho stare. I saw that he
had a whole storyline of what people had told him in the past.
Whenever his aggression came out, people would say, "Keep your
hands in your pockets," or "Turn the other cheek," or "Go get a soda
and forget it." He was from a broken home and had a history of
being isolated and rejected. His body was a tight fist of anger, and I
knew he could explode with little or no provocation.

My comment intrigued him, though, so in his tough-guy sort of way he motioned for me to say more. "Yeah," I said, "I'll teach you how to kill someone. I just want one thing from you. I want you to commit yourself to every session that I do." He raised his eyebrows a bit and then finally said, "I'll do it." For the same reason I believed he could kill someone, I believed he would come to every session. He liked to be purposeful, and he did come to every session.

In our first session together, I showed him some pressure point. It became obvious that he was so eager and excited to get his revenge on whoever it was that he had no sense of center, no sense of ground, no feeling for his body. He was fumbling around with his hands, his energy about three feet off the ground. So I said, "Wait a minute. You won't be able to kill anybody like that. We have to develop some other things first." The other things we started to develop were the bodily principles of center, ground, extension, how to organize and mobilize energy, how to blend with incoming energy. I can describe them in a few brief sentences, but it took about three months to actually teach him those principles. Every time I would show him some technique, he would fumble around, and we would go back to the bodily principles.

During this process, a change began to happen. Working very hard toward fulfilling his vendetta, this young man barely noticed that our work had slipped into an entirely new context. The best way to describe this change is to say that his attention shifted from the object of his anger back to himself. As we continued, it became clear that while he had forgotten his original motives, he became more and more immersed in the living of his excitement. Something else was beginning to take form, and it was leading him into deeper and more satisfying dimensions of himself. He was beginning to live in his body, and this provided him a context in which he could develop and work with his own experience. He began to make decisions more from what he felt and less from what he thought he should do. He had a wider range of expression, and he felt more emotions. He spoke more from his own experience and less from his peer-group code.

This wasn't always an easy process for him or me. There were times when he wanted to kill me, or I wanted to wring his neck. He would threaten to run away, and once he broke down and cried over his shifting identity. He went through everything that someone does when they psychologically die and are reborn. Our time together was full of great agonies and small victories. But as he lived more from his body, he could tell the truth about all of these things. He experienced what it meant to be responsible for himself.

Once, toward the end of our time together, we were moving and sparring around the mat in a spirit of play and cooperation, when he turned to me and said, "You know, it is easy to kill somebody. But it's more interesting to find out about myself. It's not as easy, but it's more interesting." I was blown away. In that statement, all of the edges of our three months together were rounded into a deeply satisfying confirmation. In my tough-guy sort of way, I became uncomfortable with the tears in my eyes. But they were there, and we acknowledged them.

This story underscores the importance of working with someone where they are, bringing life to their situation by simply paying attention to what is most obvious without the hindrance of a prepared sermon. If I had said to that young man, "No, no, you don't even want to think those thoughts. What you should do is keep your hands in your pockets and just keep whistling," he might have pulled his gun on me right then. His rage was the doorway to his deeper energies and desires, not something to avoid.

What is important here is the change this manchild went through to be able to say, "It's more interesting to find out about myself," and simultaneously to let go of his desire to hurt someone. The transformation he went through is one that is pivotal in personal development and evolution. It is the first step toward becoming self-healing, self-educating, and self-transforming. What happened to this young man was that he began to live in his body. Through practices and exercises, he awakened the perceptive skills of feeling and sensing. As he embodied himself he became someone, a somebody who was able to respond to life in a way that deepened and invigorated his experience. Beginning to live in his body initiated an inner dialogue that made him realize that he could be the source of his own meaning and knowledge. As his interest turned from what was outside of him toward the inner process of his own life, he became less dependent on the external situation for his identity and aliveness. Instead of only being the tough guy who was out for revenge, he became many experiences and many feelings. His responses to other people and to the environment became richer and more varied. He began to experience what Socrates meant by "Know thyself."

When we are embodied, we become learners. We can learn from situations, from our experiences, from life. If we do not live in our body, which is the seat of our experience, we are only capable of rote learning and reacting in mechanical ways. Identifying with the life of the body, and less with the demands of society and our constant caravan of thoughts and fantasies, brings us closer to our unconditioned self. This gives us the ability to genuinely respond to life.

The manchild in this story had a line that went something like this: "So and so is a jerk because he crossed me, so next time I see him, I'm going to lay him out." But as he began to inhabit his body, this line began to change. He began to feel the energy of his anger instead of its content. Instead of having to strike out with it, he was able to open himself to it. He found meaning in turning his attention toward his inner experience. He discovered a way to be with his anger different from directing it toward others. When we make such a turn in our lives, we become responsible for our actions.

Turning our attention inward in this way is not a retreat; it is an enlivening of ourself. Being with our experience, without instantly projecting it outward, gives us strength and integrity. We learn that our sense of wholeness comes from within, and we don't feel compelled to run away from our dissatisfaction. This creates an environment in which we can learn from our discontent, a ground from which to work with our pain and anxiety.

Being with ourself bodily makes it possible to participate in forming attitudes about our experience. Living in our body, we realize that we have a choice about how to relate to any given situation. We can have everything taken from us—friends, relatives, home, and status, we can be deprived of all human needs—but our attitude toward any given situation can never be taken away. If we are connected to our energy, which flows through our body, we are always left with the final choice of how we can relate to a situation. In this sense, we make the situation by the way we relate to it.

The experience of embodiment is a fundamental one. The two factors that must be understood and experienced for embodiment to take place are energy and attention. Before going on, we need to consider these.

Energy

Our energy is our aliveness. It is the stuff that creates the continuity of our life. We wake up with it, we go to bed with it, it is present in our waking and sleeping dreams. It is the river that carries the meaning and significance of our daily life. We have thoughts, images, memories, sensations, and emotions that are birthed and nurtured by this river. It is the ground from which our living emerges. "This current allies me to the rest of the world," says Thoreau. In various cultures and traditions, this energy has been variously called *ki, chi, shabd,* élan vital, *prana,* the life current. Throughout this book, the words energy and excitement mean the same thing: the ground of our existence and that which births our experience.

A primary goal in working with someone therapeutically, artistically, or educationally is to bring them into contact with their energy, that is, into the experience of their lived body. The first step is to have the person identify with what they feel, to place their attention on what is occurring in their bodily life. Attending to what we feel takes us out of our heads and into the energetic currents of our body. Living in our bodies means living in the moment. Our energy and attention weave the tapestry of who we are—bodily, emotionally, psychologically, and spiritually.

We can experience our energy in a number of ways. Energy can be the rush we feel when we are surprised or suddenly jolted. The tinglings, vibrations, and streamings that arise all over the body after a series of deep inhalations and exhalations are energy. If we clap our hands and rub them vigorously together, and then hold them about six inches apart, we feel energy as sensations in our palms. The pressure from holding our breath for as long as we can and the charge we feel after we release it are experiences of energy. The vibrations from a sustained flexion or contraction are energy. The warmth and trembling of loving someone is the energy of human contact. The pulsing around our body is our energy field. In a way, energy is nothing special, but it is the glue that binds everything together and connects us to our essential self.

Attention

In the movie *Star Wars*, there was a rather ordinary scene that jumped out at me in an unusual way. In it, Han Solo, Chewbacca, and Artoo Detoo were all standing together planning their next move, when suddenly Han Solo seemed illuminated in a way that was lacking in his companions. I asked myself, "What makes Han Solo, the human, different from the other two?" In many respects, he shares characteristics similar to his two companions. Like Artoo Detoo, the sensitive robot, he has highly developed logical and intellectual abilities; like Chewbacca, the powerful animal figure, he has the passion needed for expression and action. But Han Solo is also gifted with something else. How was he, as a human, cast differently from the animals and machines? Most obviously, he is more unpredictable than the others. But what makes this so? What is this light, this sudden change of moods, this certain receptivity to grace? It is, of course, his capacity for self-awareness. Only he can direct his attention both to the external environment and to his own internal process. It is as if he has an additional limb or organ that the others don't have—an organ of attention.

Attention is a primary ingredient in embodiment and, at the same time, the connecting thread throughout our learning and development. When we are paying attention to what we are doing, we are both learning and encouraging learning. Our attention is the rudder that guides us through the world. It gives us direction, and it connects us to the current of energy that moves us. The act of paying attention creates a quality of awakening that expands us beyond the usual dreams of prosperity and romance. Cultivating this awareness enriches our lives because it tells us who we are and how we are.

In order to embody and use ourself as a source of learning, it is necessary to identify with the life of the body. To live in our body and be aware of what we feel, touch, taste, hear, breathe, see, and think, it is necessary to shift our attention from analyzing and remembering to feeling and sensing. Bringing attention to our body vitalizes and empowers our actions. Without it our life is mechanical; we go through the motions but are not with ourself in a truly meaningful way. We can correctly form our arms around a child for a hug, for example, but if we are not paying attention, it is only a shadow of the kind of warmth that can be communicated.

Our attention is at work all of the time, probing into the world and back into ourselves. It is our natural birthright and nothing that needs to be invented. What we need to do, however, is to come into direct contact with our attention so that we can use it. When we learn how to direct our attention, we can use it to manifest meaning and wholeness.

Our attention is similar to an organ or muscle in that it functions within the biological domain and can be cultivated, nurtured, and strengthened through bodily practices. Working through the body, two principles can be understood with respect to the organ of attention.

The first principle is that the attention can be directed. It is, in other words, flexible and not confined to a specific sense organ. In fact, it is attention that imbues the sense organs with presence and vitality. Like a powerful laser beam, the organ of attention can be directed in all possible directions, within ourself and outside of ourself. To experience this, bring your attention to your hands and fingers as you hold this book. As you do, a tremendous amount of information will come to you about the texture of the paper, the weight of the book, the pressure of your fingers as they hold the book. Now direct your attention to the sounds in the room or in other rooms, and a whole new package of information will come to you through the audio channel. Yet your hands remain holding the book, touching the pages.

Now take your attention to your memory of the last meal you ate. As your attention probes your memory, highlights of that meal will appear, perhaps even with tactile and taste sensations. Now come back to the experience of holding the book. The sounds of the room remain, the memories remain, but we are now focused on something different. It is as though we have a channel selector that can focus on a multitude of stations. This power of directing attention is key in embodying ourselves. By integrating this capacity, we have a way of bringing ourself back to the experience of the life of the body and anchoring ourself in the present moment.

The second principle is that attention can vitalize or devitalize a situation. This is because it magnetizes energy, and where we place our attention, energy will follow. By turning the attention to a specific bodily function, we can gather information about that function and also initiate a change in that area and ultimately in our behavior. Charles Darwin said, "Attention or conscious concentration on almost any part of the body produces some direct physical effect on it." This can be experienced by focusing on a bodily pain. If your attention concentrates on this pain, you will find that the pain is not static and unchanging but something dynamic and moving, and the power of your attention can become a key factor in working with and lessening the pain. By focusing our attention inward, we can gain a better understanding of the numerous signals our body transmits concerning health and well-being. To find out if it is time to eat, to use a simple example, we can focus on our stomach instead of the clock or some idea about the "right" time to eat.

In this moment, take your attention inside and see if you can contact your heart. Can you feel where it is, its rhythm, its power, the messages it may be sending you? If you allow your attention to reside with your heart, without anything special in mind about what should happen, you will find that your pulse rate will soon change. It will most likely become slower and more rhythmic. And as the heart opens more fully, the chest will soften and fill with warmth, affecting our relationship with others and with our immediate world.

The organ of attention has enormous possibilities for healing and learning. When you find yourself engulfed in thoughts about an upsetting situation, for example, see if you can redirect your attention from the thoughts to the breath. Don't try to do anything with your breath; just be with it, attend to it, soak in it with your attention. If the upsetting thoughts return, go back to the feelings and sensations of your breath as it moves along your belly and torso or at your nostrils. This is not to ignore or repress certain feelings or thoughts, but rather an alternative way to work with anxiety.

If we place our attention on that which is lifegiving and creative, that part of us will be nourished. If we place our attention on negativity, that will be cultivated. Nietzsche said it in a particularly interesting way: "If we look too long into the abyss we will fall into it."

Here is another simple exercise to illustrate the principles and uses of attention. Sit comfortably with your eyes open and let your attention gaze out a window. Now bring the attention to the window frame. Now bring it to an object near to you. Now bring it to the sensations of your feet on the floor, now to the rhythm of your breath, now deep inside of you to someplace that you would call your core. As you shifted your attention, the objects remained, but the power of attention illuminated and energized each one in turn. All of the objects are existing at the same time, but it is our attention that brings them into the foreground of our experience. In the same way, we can illuminate the embodied state by using our attention to identify with our body instead of our memories and fantasies.

Paying attention to what we are doing provides a spaciousness that allows self-inquiry to take place. With our attention, we can literally open ourselves to participate in something that is larger than the boundaries we are normally accustomed to. Through an ongoing practice of paying attention, we can begin to contact an intelligence that is deep enough to be the source of our learning and precise enough to show us how we learn. This awareness is the basis for learning and transformation.

One of the best ways to cultivate the organ of attention is to set aside some part of the day to practice. A way to do this is to sit comfortably in a chair or on a pillow with your eyes either open or closed. Keep your attention on your breath, either at the abdomen as it rises and falls or as it enters and leaves the nose. When you wander off into thought or memory, simply bring your attention back to the breath. Doing this daily, for either fifteen minutes, half an hour, or an hour, will strengthen the organ of attention and increase your ability to return to the embodied state.

Living in our bodies has a sort of exotic sound about it, like going to Club Mediterranean for a holiday or setting up camp on some charming beach. But, in truth, living in our bodies is perhaps the most fundamental part of our existence, and it happens right here. I use the term "living" body to distinguish it from the anatomical body. Everyone knows they have a body and can name its parts, but it is the living body where we actually experience our aliveness through emotions, sensations, temperatures, actions, and energetic states. By living in our body we can participate in our life, and by doing this we can learn from our experience.

A major goal of working with someone somatically, then, is to help them to live in their body. The essential step in beginning to do this is to bring our attention to the sensations we feel. They may be hot, cold, hard, soft, heavy, light, rough, or smooth, and to feel them is to begin to connect with the life that is in the body. Out of this initial connection, we may feel such emotions as joy, happiness, anger, or sadness. Or we may feel energetic states like flowings, vibrations, pulsations, streamings, auras, or currents. When we place our attention in our body we begin to feel, and our feeling connects us to our energy. Our energy then informs us of our direction and meaning in life. If we respond from our energy, we are responding from that part of ourselves that is least conditioned. If we act from our energy, and not from our ideas, social images, or what others expect, we feel enriched with genuine expression and life.

To perform mechanical exercises that strengthen the body or conform it to an external image of attractiveness is not necessarily living in the body. Nor is it the development of a technique that intensifies certain emotions, nor a method that subdues us into calmness and neutrality. Rather it is feeling and living from the current of life that animates all things.

According to the notion of living in our body right posture is born through an inner feeling of wellness and wholeness, not through manipulation of the tissues or a series of mechanical exercises. Early in my training, when I was concerned with aligning bodies structurally, a certain client taught me something very important. He was a bright, interesting man who made his living teaching philosophy. Because his posture was characterized by a head that hung in front of his torso somewhat like a vulture's the work focused around his neck and shoulders. After I spent much time stretching and restructuring the tissues in his neck and shoulders, he regained the anatomical flexibility to align his head on top of his shoulders and to fill out his chest. After one of these sessions, he was able to stand and view the world from a more upright position. He could feel his legs under him, and he enjoyed the increased feeling in his chect and stomach. I felt successful and he felt satisfied. But a half a block away from the office his shoulders began to round, his head dropped down and forward, and his chest caved in. He again became someone who was probing the world with his lurking head while tying off the rest of his body. Later, when asked about this reverse metamorphosis, he simply replied that he did not feel like himself without his head that far forward. It was traditional for a philosophy professor to have that kind of posture. This helped me understand that living in our bodies comes from an inner feeling and not from movements or postures that are mechanically correct.

Living in the body can be seen as having three different stages. The first is *body as feedback*, which is when we direct our attention to a certain area of our body—a shoulder, our jaw, feet, stomach—and we embody the sensations that we feel there. After we learn to do this, we can then use these bodily parts as feedback for certain emotional, structural, and functional states. Our tense shoulders, for example, may tell us we are afraid, or our clenched fists may tell us we are anxious and holding back, or we may realize that our bad knee actually originates in the way we squeeze our lower back. In this stage we are definitely in a relationship with our body, but we are not yet living in it totally. The body is like a new friend that we are getting to know.

The next stage is *body as being*. At this point, the entire body becomes a state of attention. We do not necessarily concentrate on a single point or part, but rather experience ourself as a living wholeness. We begin to embody our actions and values. This is when we are truly able to relax and in doing so we exude an energetic presence.

The third stage is *body as path*. In this stage, we begin to develop such abilities as clairsentience, which is bodily intuition and healing power. We have integrated the principles of grounding, centering, blending, and energetic perception in such a way as to use them in our social, emotional, and spiritual lives. At this point we are at one with the energy that moves through us. We are both one with our body and at the same time, more than our body. We can identify with ourself and others as pulsating, magnetic energy fields.

These three stages overlap and are not so clearly defined in the living of them, but as a map they are helpful in understanding what it means to live in the body. A man I will call Brett went through many of these stages over the four years he was involved in bodywork, therapy, and aikido.

Brett

Brett was a huge man who worked in the building trade, and his strength was in his barrel chest and thick, sinewy arms. He had a front that was gruff, knowing, and independent, and he had sort of an "I don't need anybody for anything" attitude. His chin, which jutted out like the prow of a ship, said "Go ahead and try it. I dare you." But for a huge man, he took up very little space. He squeezed himself into the chair, held his legs tightly together, and spoke to the air about a foot in front of him. His legs, in contrast to his upper body, were spindly and taut. His feet and toes were like claws that gripped the earth. He lumbered about like a sullen, watchful giant. Brett was distant, but he somehow gave the feeling of wanting to join, to be included. He had the urge to grow, but his heavily armored body kept him caged.

Although Brett had the image of himself as being fit and active, mostly because his job kept him outside and physically active, the quality of light usually associated with health and an emerging presence was lacking in his tissues. His skin, pulled taut across his large frame, lacked vibrancy and color. Much of Brett's excitement gathered in his eyes and forehead. His eyes were a brilliant blue, and they guarded against any entry into who he was by staring fixedly out. He thought this made him look intense and interested, but it was obvious that he saw very little. Only small breaths came into his massive chest, and at the end of each in-breath he always, if only for a moment held his breath and compressed the entire length of his torso, from his neck to his genitals.

As he sat before me I thought, "This is a twelve-year-old boy in a grown-up's body. Behind all of those muscles is a terrified kid." Despite his voice, which sounded like he was reading a train schedule, and his white knuckles gripping the chair, Brett said he felt "just fine." How Brett thought of himself and how he actually was seemed very different.

Brett came to work on himself mostly at the urging of his wife and business associates. He said that he had reached a "flat spot" in his life, which he later revealed to mean increasing migraine headaches, lack of sexual interest, diminishing job productivity, and an expensive cocaine habit. Brett was thirty-four at that time and had been married for ten years, with no children. He was born in the midwest, went to a small midwestern college on an athletic scholarship, came to the West Coast with the navy, and followed in his father's footsteps to becoming a building contractor.

In the first three sessions, we talked and basically got to know each other. In the fourth session, Brett was interested in doing some bodywork. I asked him to simply lie down and be as open as possible to what came up. The thing that was most obvious about Brett was that he wasn't really lying on the mat at all. The long muscles along his spine were taut cables, his big chest was puffed up like a held bladder, and his arms and hands were pushing down, as if he were trying to keep himself away from the ground. His bulging eyes, set in a battle against blinking, looked as if he were a thousand yards down the road. He allowed very little breath to come in and he carefully measured each out-breath. As he narrowed himself in this way, pulling away from the possibility of any contact, a gray green shadow tinted his complexion. It was as if he had covered himself with a protective shroud that dampened the life in and around him. When asked how he felt, he said, "Fine." Again there was this huge chasm between how he was and how he wanted to be seen. It was the same as the contradiction between his overbound, muscular torso and his small, underdeveloped legs. Brett had somehow convinced himself that life in this self-imposed coffin was the ticket to strength and well-being. He seemed to equate stiffness and rigidity with poise and manhood. In reality, he wasn't living in his body at all, but only in his idea of himself. Brett's conditioned tendency was to squeeze his chest, throat, and eyes and to act the part of a "good boy." His rhythm of excitment was to overemphasize the stage of containment.

After a while, I gently touched Brett on the chin. His jaw looked like it was chewing on a bit. We drew his attention to this and the fact that the body is designed so the teeth do not have to touch. He learned that if he found himself always biting down, he was probably holding his jaw too tight. He also learned that a tightly held jaw can cause headaches, eyestrain, and even earaches. Brett was basically out of touch with the tight grip he held around his mouth and jaw. Only when I repeatedly touched his chin was he able to feel this holding. A few times I asked him to bite even harder, to consciously enact the squeezing and tension in his jaw. This brought more awareness to the area, and it increased his ability to locate the tension and then to let go of it.

When he did release his jaw, his eyes would soften, his chest would momentarily relax, and deeper breath would follow. What was happening, in effect, was that Brett was beginning to embody this part of himself. He began to live in his jaw, and he began to experience what was happening there. This was the beginning of Brett's living in his body and using himself as his own source of information. It was also the first time in a long time that he had consciously turned his attention to what he was feeling. Repeatedly touching Brett's chin to remind him to let go of his jaw, and having him do a few exercises between sessions helped him discover how much he held in his jaw. This gave him a growing awareness of his biting down and its effects on his teeth and eyes. A month after this discovery, he made the connection between his migraines and the clenched jaw. Two weeks after that session, he connected his jaw to an emotional repression. A series of insights and perceptions like this will commonly lead from one into another in working bodily.

In the session that he discovered the emotional history of his clenched jaw, we were focusing on the feeling and attitude in his face. Suddenly a memory was evoked in which Brett saw "my father telling me, many times, as sort of a teaching to 'keep your mouth shut and look alert'. He didn't even really say it in a mean or admonishing way, but he said it a lot, like something that would be useful in life. A way to get ahead I suppose."

He wove this memory into his present life by experimenting with different facial attitudes, gestures, sounds, and movements that gave him a feeling for how he shaped his life with a "shut mouth."

In the next session he said, "I realized this week that this whole thing with my jaw makes it almost impossible for me to say anything directly. In my home town, keeping your mouth shut and looking alert was what a good boy did, and I'm still doing it." Brett's face held a curiosity that was mixed with both anger and the relief that often comes from an emotional discovery. "Why do I do this to my-self?" he wondered.

Following his curiosity, Brett traced this question back to his wanting approval from his father. He looked at how he played the approval game by being a good boy. He played it long enough and sincere enough that it became a habit, in other words, a fixed atti-tude in his muscles. He then saw how he became so addicted to the habit that he didn't even notice when he wasn't getting what he orig-inally wanted—approval. Somewhere along the line, maybe when he was about fourteen, Brett decided to go about being a man in his father's eyes. The ground of feeling and desire that he had denied in order to gain approval was what now lay fallow in him.

Although he built the correct forms to get approval—he devel-oped a strong, muscular chest and arms, was an excellent athlete and an outstanding naval officer, had a beautiful wife and a business like his father's—he never really lived in any of these bodies. He was someplace else, acting out his "good boy" image without feeling who he was or what he wanted. Then when all of his accomplishments were added up and there still wasn't approval or satisfaction, Brett became more and more sullen. He suddenly didn't know what he wanted or what was important, but something was ticking in him. The bad boy was pushing through: his legs were pissed off for car-rying that big front for so long, his head ached from thoughts and controlling strategies, his heart disappeared under the tomb of his rigid chest, his addiction switched to cocaine, and he became diffi-cult to live with.

As these feelings and insights began to surface, Brett began to get angry about them. Now that his jaw had less control, he would begin to say things that surprised him. He would shout, "Fuck you, Dad!" or "I resent my damn construction company." When he first started to spontaneously express these things, he would often flip to the good boy, who would be self-critical, or he would deal with his angry feelings with false compassion. He would say, "My father treated me well; I have no right to be angry," or "He didn't know what he was doing. I understand what he had to do." Brett had com-passion, but its genuineness was suffocating under layers of anger and frustration. He was afraid that if he wasn't a good boy during these times his rage might become as big as himself, and he would break the furniture. He was big and he was angry, yet there was a basic sense of caring that was natural to him. In his growing up, caring meant being a sissy, and Brett didn't want to be a sissy—he wanted to be like his dad. Yet it was the quality of caring in this large, rough man that made Brett unique and approachable.

During these sessions, I encouraged Brett to experience his feelings of denial, care, and anger as felt, bodily experiences. Out of fear, he would resist by changing the subject, talking about and rationalizing his feelings, or becoming the phony good boy who understood. He would then be directed back to what he felt in his body. This helped him replace his opinions and judgments about himself with concrete bodily experiences. In his initial experiences of feeling his body, Brett would either have a wonderful sense of warmth and well-being or would be swept into terror and panic. Having controlled his world for so long, it was overwhelming for him to be washed by the tides of sensation and feeling. But Brett saw this as a challenge, and he slowly began to move into his body. By bringing his perceptions and feelings into forms of gesturing, sounding, pushing, kicking, and rhythms of breath, he slowly began to trust his excitement. It was shaky new ground, but Brett was now starting to experience his body, and it was telling him an interesting story about himself. His body became the barometer of his feelings, desires, denials, and potentials, and he wanted more.

In a session a few months later, Brett was lying on his back and experiencing the breath in his stomach. As he slowly began to drop lower and deeper into his body, his abdomen began to soften and round as he inhaled. His chest began to relax and surrender its puffed-up defense. He began to breathe more deeply than in any previous session, and he began to let go into the floor. It looked as though a weight had just dropped off Brett, and he became both quiet and alert. Then out of nowhere a laugh began to well up from deep inside of him. His whole body shook with this laughter, and tears flowed from his eyes. Soon the sound of his laughter filled me and the room. Brett was feeling himself deeply, and it gave him great satisfaction.

His laughing subsided, and he became quiet again. His brow swiftly knit into a fierce knot, his breathing became shallow and fast, and his eyes darted furtively around the room. He said that he was anxious and that he felt worried about the uncontrollable laughter.

He recalled his father criticizing him when he was a young boy for laughing uncontrollably. Brett also remarked that his father was a very rigid, disciplined, and successful man whom he had never seen laugh.

When asked what it felt like to feel worried, he began to explain his thoughts which took him away from his experience. He was running from his discomfort, but he wasn't able to leave it behind. It tailed him like a mean little dog, and he couldn't quite shake it off with his hurried explanation. Working bodily, our interest is in how worry feels and not in what it thinks. I told him that we might work with his mental associations later, but now we needed to find out how and where he felt his worry and anxiety. This would establish a ground from which he could later explore other dimensions of himself.

He was willing to do this, and he began to experience and verbalize the way he was squeezing his eyes and forehead (and probably his brain), holding his breath, and pinching himself at the diaphragm. As his attention began to connect with those parts of his body, his experience began to change. His anxiety began to form into anger and resentment, and this took the form of excitement in his shoulders and arms. Whereas he would have repressed this feeling before, Brett now allowed it to come to form. With his voice, hands, arms, and legs, he fought for his right to laugh, to experience satisfaction, to let go of the controls that he adopted from his father. He slammed his powerful arms into the mat and roared. Brett's rage turned to weeping that came around again to laughter and then to joy.

This was a turning point in Brett's work. Participating in his embodied experience, Brett discovered how he could release habitual patterns through his body. This also made him less afraid of his emotions. He discovered how his excitement and emotional character could change form and flow from one expression into another. It was a relief for him to know that he wouldn't necessarily be caught in one emotion.

In physically recreating his process of holding, Brett experienced where and how he constricted himself. This gave him a reference point from which he could experience letting go. He then began to see how he could use himself to gather information and take it into action. By contacting his muscles, weight, balance, and movements, he could feel how he was making his life "flat." He discovered that when he felt himself deeply he satisfied a very old and profound need. Later he would cognitively understand that his father's image did not necessarily have to be his own, but first he experienced the difference between discursive thinking/analysis/memory and embodiment. This distinction between feeling and thinking gave Brett a sense of responsibility that enriched his life. It gave him the opportunity to be touched and moved by his excitement instead of moving into a set pattern of reaction based on an old memory. By contacting his body, Brett began to understand on a deeper level who he was.

In the months that followed, Brett worked with his ability to tolerate his excitement as it manifested itself in feelings, actions, and satisfaction. The word "tolerate" is used in the sense of being with, not in the sense of putting up with. In other words, when he would restrict certain feelings or responses because of old belief patterns, he would continue to return his attention to the feelings as a way of increasing his capacity for feeling. In this way, he recognized the old patterns but emphasized the new excitement.

When he began to work with his legs and grounding, for example, I would place my hands on his thighs, calves, and feet and ask him to come into that area with his attention. Sometimes the touch would be light and at other times the work would be deep into the tissues. When he would retreat into his head, I would encourage him to return to his legs by placing his attention on the sensation of the touch. In other instances, I would move his legs and joints while he paid attention to the movement. In each case, what was important was that he take his attention to that part of his leg. If some emotional content or memory was evoked, that would be the ground of the work, but at the most basic level he was living deeper and deeper in the experience of his legs. To live in our bodies we must contact the feeling dimension of ourselves, and this was the foundation of Brett's work.

After a while, Brett went through a phase where the work took him to standing. This helped him feel his legs as mobility, ground, and support. He would take his attention to his legs and feel how his weight could be transferred through his hip, knee, and ankle joints, and then to the earth beneath his feet. In these sessions, he would walk and jump in order to experience his legs as support and as way to mobilize his excitement. As he embodied his legs more, he found a greater strength and flexibility in them. He discovered ways of holding his ground without being rigid. He also uncovered ways of mobility that were relaxed and at the same time grounded and supportive.

Focusing on his grounding, Brett also learned to kick and push with his legs and feet. As he allowed his excitement to form into these movements, his hips, legs, and feet became alive with a spontaneous assortment of movements: stamping, kicking, pushing, pedaling, scissoring, and stomping. Accompanying these were various emotional states that were expressed by sounds of anger, joy, effort, resistance, rage, desire, and laughter. It was reminiscent of how infants will kick, punch, flail, frog kick, and scissor with their legs to act out feelings of hunger, elation, fatigue, and just pure enjoyment at being alive, like tadpoles kicking and swimming toward evolution. These exercises also taught Brett how his excitement could form, be expressed, and then re-form into a new expression.

Throughout most of his life, Brett had relied on his massive chest and powerful arms as his ground. But maintaining his defensive posture and high center of gravity took constant effort. It also took very little pressure for this ground to give way, and when it did he would either fall into a depression, explode into tantrums of violence, or, as he finally did, turn to drugs. But as he slowly began to use his legs, breath, and vision as a grounding force, his overbound upper body began to relax; he then began to find interest and pleasure in unexpected things. As his investment with his macho, "I can go it alone" began to loosen, his sensitivity and caring began to emerge. He began carving and sculpting, which led him to an artistic community that gathered in studios instead of bars. With his new reserves of energy, he began landscaping the houses he built. As he began to live in his body, he accepted and trusted himself more, and his longing for contact flowed into people and creative interests.

As Brett began to live more from the experience of his body, he began to find more satisfaction in the living and expression of his life. His migraine headaches were nonexistent, he hadn't used cocaine for almost two years, and he was becoming more and more intimate in his relationships. At this point, Brett had embodied himself enough to have the skills to use his body as a feedback system for knowing who he was structurally, functionally, and emotionally.

Because Brett had met his goals for a healthier and more productive life, we were at a frontier in the work. He felt satisfied with his accomplishments, but he also wanted to continue working with himself and to connect with others who had the same interests. In his words, "I want to keep growing and working on myself. I feel like I'm finally at a place where I can actually move ahead. I need a way to bring all of this into my life. Now I feel like all my insights and awarenesses are the same one told in different ways. I need to put them in action." In some way Brett felt stuck, even with all of his revelations and discoveries. Even though he saw a lot, he was unable to translate many of his perceptions into appropriate action and behavior. This marked a new stage in his work. At this point, after working with Brett for two years, I encouraged him to take up a bodily discipline. He had started doing sitting meditation as a way to work with his body and attention, but he knew it was necessary, if he wanted to continue on his journey, that he participate in some bodily endeavor that involved other people.

After some discussion and trying T'ai Chi, yoga, and running, Brett joined the aikido dojo. He preferred the contact of aikido, he enjoyed the crowd that trained at the dojo, and he found himself enjoying the new skills of rolling, falling, and working with his aggression. But what stood out most for Brett was the realization that his knowing and insights had little value while he was on the mat. He soon discovered that when someone was punching, grabbing, kicking, or moving at him, it really didn't matter what he knew or how he verbalized it. What mattered was whether he could embody his knowledge. He now needed to act from the information that he was receiving through the text of his body. If someone was punching at him, for example, it was no longer enough for him to realize that he should be centered. He was now in an arena in which he had to *be* centered. Aikido became a perfect laboratory for Brett to experiment with transforming his perceptions and feelings into action.

As Brett became more involved in aikido, we met every other week for a while and then only once a month before we terminated our client/therapist relationship. But during this overlap, there were significant changes in his levels of embodiment. First of all, he began to learn how to open up his focus. Using his entire body as a state of attention, he learned the skill of moving and acting from a center. After about three months of aikido, he was also learning how to truly relax. It was not only the deeper letting go when he would lie down and breathe; he was now able to experience relaxation as he sat, conversed, and walked down the street. This too was a result of his open focus and using his entire body as a state of attention.

A year and a half later, Brett's body had changed along with his personality. He was softer and rounder, and there was an overall sense of his being closer to the ground. He had a new aura of sensitivity and power. Being more fluid and more in touch with himself and others, Brett was tapping a source of power that was much deeper and much more effective than his old forward, muscle-bound approach.

He said that he was still a building contractor but that his main interest was the volunteer work he was doing at a halfway house for runaway children. He discovered that he had talent for working with children, and he taught them aikido. He said he could track their needs and moods in an uncanny way. "I can sense their ki and know instinctively how they will react to certain situations and events," he said. This was the development of clairsentience, which is bodily intuition or perception, and it was becoming a path for him to connect deeper with himself and other people. Mostly there was a new and fresh meaning in his life, and it was rooted in the experience of his body and energy. Living in his body had become an ongoing path for Brett.

Once we have the ability to live from the life of our body, we can begin to tap into its wisdom and potential. In the next chapter, we will learn various bodily practices and energetic states to assist us in times of confusion and transition. These are forms that we can use in order to move through change and overcome obstacles in our everyday situations.

THE ANATOMY OF CHANGE

"The important thing is this: To be able at any moment to sacrifice what we are for what we could become."
Charles Dubois

In 1975, I experienced four major changes within a period of eight months. I fractured my arm in two places and was in a cast from shoulder to wrist for over two months; I spent a summer in Japan studying aikido; I went through a major reorientation in my professional life; and I ended an eight-year relationship. As these changes reached across my physical, emotional, social, professional, and cultural life, I was required to reorganize myself on all levels. It was a confusing, painful, and exciting time. I felt like I was suddenly asked to play in a game in which I didn't know the rules or even have a program that could tell me who was playing. But in ways that I was unaware of at the time, I was being provided with tremendous material and insight in to the process of change and its relationship to learning.

When my cast was removed, I began juggling and playing the flute in order to regain coordination in my injured arm. Never having juggled or played a musical instrument before, I was on virgin soil. As I began to exercise my arm and myself in new ways, I not only learned new skills and a new use of my arm, I also became interested in how I learned. My excitement was not just in what I was learning, or in the exhilaration of learning and new health, but in *how* I was learning.

Later, my entry into a foreign culture, the transition of ending an intimate relationship, and the confusion around major changes in my professional life all became intertwined with the rehabilitation of my broken arm, which became ground for learning and growth. In this disintegration and upheaval, I experienced that the steps I went through in learning to reuse my broken arm were the same steps I went through in my emotional, cultural, and psychological changes. I experienced that our bodily life and our psychological, emotional, and social life are somehow all linked together. This notion of learning through the body, and its connection to other areas of life, became a consuming interest.

This period taught me that just as change can be a condition for learning, learning also involves change. Learning, in fact, is a process of change. In order to learn, we must to a certain degree let go of who we think we are and what we think we know. This transition, from what we are to what we can become, is where we learn and where we have the potential of seeing *how* we learn.

The idea of change being natural, or even creative, goes against our social conditioning. However obvious and fundamental change may be in our life, our culture and educational system do little to instruct us in how to work through transitions. Because of the upheaval that often accompanies change, we are expected and taught to view change as a calamity. Except for assuming the image of the good, brave soldier with a stiff upper lip or of the noble martyr who becomes the crushed victim, or for irresponsibly covering our eyes until the change is over, we have few skills for moving through change. Consequently, various ills and diseases associated with stress and anxiety are epidemic in industrialized nations. Yet it is possible to accept change and the upsets that may arise out of it as an opportunity to move ahead, to let go of something that is no longer useful for our journey.

Because our educational system emphasizes the teaching of concepts, we are given a rather static or fixed sense of what is real. With the accent on conceptual learning, we are never educated into the how of living through change. It is a fundamental flaw in our educational system that we are never truly educated to deal with the living process of life. We are taught the language and concepts of society, in order to function in society, but rarely are we taught the language of movement, of life, of moving through the unknown. At the same time, our traditions and institutions over the past fifty years have changed in ways that cause them to have little to offer us in terms of managing our life transitions. To fill this void, we can turn toward the living body to help usher us through the many changes and up-heavals that we go through in a lifetime, or in a day. By honoring our bodily and energetic life, we can begin to understand something not only about our individual process but also about the principles inherent in change.

It is possible, in other words, to learn how different bodily and energetic shapes, rhythms, movements, and sensations can guide and inform us through our transitions. These bodily messages be-come a living language that can direct us when we find our world falling apart. This language signals us when it is time to express our feelings and when it is time to take our feelings inside to embrace and know intimately; it tells us when we are blocking ourselves and when we are free and unhindered; it teaches how our muscles, like ourself, may work in a creative tension to make the appropriate ges-ture.

By working through our body, it is possible to creatively guide ourselves through transitions, through learning situations, and through times of fear and anxiety. This bodily way of working through obstacles is what I call the anatomy of change. It is about letting go of the old so that the new may take form. The following is a metaphor for the anatomy of change.

Imagine yourself sitting at a table holding a cup. The cup rep-resents the quantity of potential, or energy or responsibility, that you are able to integrate into your life at this particular moment. After being with this cup of yourself for some time, you notice that there is a quart container on the table. The quart represents the possibility of even more energy, responsibility, and love. You begin to recognize that the quart is within your reach. Since you have explored the lim-its of your cup, you feel an urge to move toward the quart. To re-main with only the cup of yourself is no longer tolerable. You make the choice to reach across the table and take the "more" of yourself. Realizing it is impossible to hold both cup and quart at the same time, you put the cup down and extend toward the quart. Panic! Part way into your reach, you realize that the comfort and familiarity of the cup are gone, and you haven't yet touched the quart. There is nothing. There are no boundaries, there is no known sense of identity or self—only empty space, a strange new land. You are thrust into fear and doubt.

At this point, what usually happens is we quickly retreat to that which is known: the cup. It is safe, familiar, and easily handleable. Or we contract, frozen in our fear of the unknown. Somehow our system of education never teaches us how to navigate these open waters, to trust ourself and our energy in times of change. We need to rediscover the passage between the cup and quart of ourselves.

The bodily skills of moving through change can be applied to any change we may be going through or to the learning of any new skill. They are skills that can be used when we are overtaken by our confusion and neurosis, and they offer the possibility of getting away from our conditioned reactions to change and of revealing "what is" about who we are and where we are going. Moving through change is an organic process of healing and education that results in a deepening involvement and commitment to the living of our life. It concerns itself with the space between the "cup and the quart": the transition place between giving up the old and the forming of the new. This process is one of trusting the wisdom of our energy, especially in times of pressure, conflict, and new input.

Moving through change has five stages: center, ground, entering and blending, skillful action (positive/extension, receptive/allowing, relaxation, timing), and union. These stages, like segments of a bridge, build on one another to make a whole. They can also be thought of as parts of an unfolding telescope, which can be effective only if each part is complete and built on the previous segment. In this way, all five stages become an ongoing living process. This means that when one stage is consolidated and integrated, it is not necessarily left behind. It unfolds as a support for the other segments in order that the whole may be perceived. It is much like protoplasm, which forms itself into a structure with boundaries in order that it may acquire mobility and continue to grow.

These stages are simple and direct in the doing though seldom taught or used as foundations for learning. Although I have arranged them in linear fashion and connected them to a specific insight, they are useful simply when they are useful. For, in fact, these stages are also states of being. To think that they can be used only in certain circumstances, or only in a certain sequence, is artificial and unrealistic. Each state can be important in any situation, at any time.

Each state also has a degree of power in it. If we are seduced by that power, chances are we will stop at that particular stage. But this is contrary to the nature of change, and holding on to a certain stage, overdeveloping a state, or claiming its power as our own can stop our growth. If this happens, we become rigid and have to expend a great deal of energy defending our position.

Keep in mind that although I am describing bodily forms and practices, they represent states of being that are applicable to all aspects of life. The experience of center in the body, for example, can through practice be passed into our intellectual, emotional, social, and spiritual life. This refers us back to our original premise, that in working through the body, we can contact the totality of our being. So keep in mind that each state, though described as a bodily practice, has value and effectiveness in all areas of our existence.

Center

Center is the starting place in the continuum of moving through change. In many respects it cannot be emphasized enough, because without it there can be very little genuine movement. Center is like the eyepiece of the telescope: it establishes a focus and place of departure for the entire spectrum of somatic learning. If, at any point in our learning and transition we feel stuck, we must return to center. Center establishes an openness and a willingness to see what is happening. We don't necessarily have to agree with the situation, but we must be willing to see what is actually happening in order to work through our fear. To be willing to see "what is" is a formidable task. Center creates the environment in which this willingness can take form.

In times of crisis and transition, we are usually filled with ideas and opinions about what is happening or what should happen. We are in a state of reaction. If we don't have a center or a place to orient around, we are swept away, along with any possibility of openness and willingness. If we are willing to experience our situation as it is, without getting ensnared in our conditioned tendency, there is a possibility to learn and grow from our experience. From a centered stance we need to ask ourselves, "Am I willing and open to the situation as it is?"

Center is a basic bodily presence, and it is on this presence that the other bodily states are built. It is a bodily and energetic base camp. When we discover ourselves drifting helplessly in our projections and memories, center is a place to anchor. Instead of floating away in our fantasies or being devoured by our thoughts, we can focus on the pulsations, temperatures, movements, and weight of our bodily form. In a sense this is a coming home, where we can begin to trust what we feel and sense.

From the somatic perspective of the lived body, this coming home is defined by the physical dimensions of the body itself. If center is the place we operate from, then the entire living body is center. It is formed by the somatic dimensions inherent in all living things: length, width, and depth. As living forms, we have a top and a bottom, a left and a right, a front and a back. From this point of view, to center is to experience our body in a total way. Center, in this sense, is the experience of ourselves in weight, time, and space.

A number of traditional Eastern disciplines define specific centers within the body. Zen Buddhism and the Japanese martial arts, for example, describe the *hara*, a point two inches below the navel, as the center of gravity and the place where *ki* (or "life energy") originates. The Sufis draw attention to the heart center as the place to develop compassion and devotion. The Indian spiritual texts describe the Third Eye, a point between and just above the physical eyes, as the center for spiritual transcendence. These centers evoke specific qualities of energy and are powerful points of focus for developing ourselves. Although the somatic notion is that the living body itself is center, it is often helpful to use *hara* as an orientation for developing center.

The concept of center is not a new one, but very few people understand it as an experience. The idea of center and the embodied experience of center are two different things. What most of us do is take an intellectual understanding of center and then try to act a certain way. The *idea* of center usually manifests itself as aloofness, detachment, rigidity, or some form of narcissism. From this idea, an attitude is shaped within the musculature, and soon we see a person who is thinking the idea of center but not experiencing it. Center, in other words, is more than an idea. It is an embodied experience that can be felt, and that can be used as a way to focus, learn, and move through transitions. It is also something that can be developed through practice.

Here is a simple exercise to bring center into the lived realm (Figure 1). Stand comfortably with your feet shoulder-width apart, one foot in front of the other. Have the back foot at about a 50-degree angle to the front foot (Figure 1a), and face your head in the

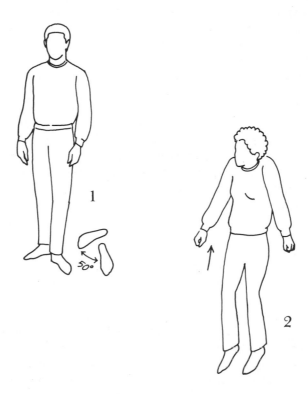

direction of the front foot. The knees are slightly bent and the arms
hang relaxed to the side. With your attention begin to sweep the
bodily dimensions: feel the contact your feet have to the floor, feel
your legs accepting the weight of your torso, feel the back straight
without stiffness, and keep your chest and stomach relaxed and soft,
your vision open and accepting, and your weight evenly distributed
between the left and right legs. Stand in a total way that is balanced
from front to back, left to right, and top to bottom. To go through
this process and experience this description as an embodied state is
to feel yourself as a living center.

Now stand as high as possible on your toes and bring your
shoulders up to your ears (Figure 2). Puff up your chest, suck in
your belly, and walk around the room in this way. This posture rep
resents being off center. It is a position and attitude of being high,
off balance, lost in thoughts, and constricted. Now take a step back

and slowly lower yourself back into center, your feet coming firmly to the earth, your legs accepting the weight of your torso, your abdomen relaxing, your chest softening, your shoulders hanging relaxed as if they were on coat hangers, your back straight. Connect with an overall sense of alertness and aliveness. What do the structural dimensions of center feel like? What is the experience of the internal state of center? What is the process of recognizing being off center, coming into center, and being with center? This simple exercise can be done over and over until you begin to feel comfortable with the passage into the embodied and felt sense of center.

It is important to remember that center is a state of being that is not confined to a certain posture or a constantly held image. Because it is through the body that we are working, the state of center is always available, despite our posture, physical handicaps, or environment. Ultimately, center is an inner subjective state that is manifested through the body. In other words, we can relate to center from any number of positions or actions. Lying down, sitting, carrying a sleeping child, washing the dishes, or driving a car can all be done from center. Being with center is an attitude toward ourself, and this attitude, formed by the boundaries of our lived body, is one in which we feel bodily present to ourself and our situation.

It is not that we have to find our center and then maintain it at all costs. Center is more of a reference point to return to, so we can relate to our life situations in a complete way. When Morihei Uyeshiba, the founder of aikido, was asked if he ever lost his balance, he replied, "Yes, all the time, but I regain it so fast that you do not see me lose it." The state of center is a doorway, a place to begin feeling our deeper urges, our possibilities in the world, the expansiveness of our excitement, and also our need to be nourished in quiet, contained ways. Because it is not an end in itself, it is not necessary to spend forever perfecting center.

Now again use the centering exercise to center yourself, and then have a partner press firmly and steadily on your chest. This pressure is much like the grab that was described in Chapter Three. If you are thinking about center (or anything else for that matter) or only have the idea of center and not the embodied experience, you will find yourself tipping backward like an inverted pyramid (Figure 3). It is almost as if the weight of the thought has made your head heavier and more lopsided than the rest of your body. If you experience being centered as an embodied experience, however, neither will you be pushed over nor will you lean forward to buttress against

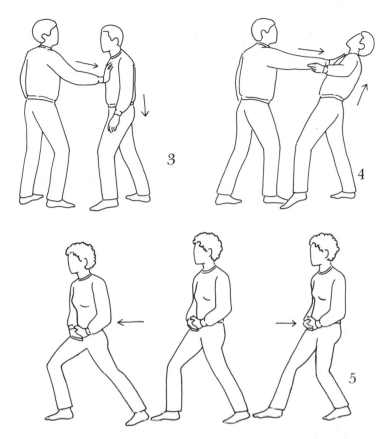

the push (Figure 4). You will feel a sense of rootedness and at the same time a softness, or flexibility. To experience yourself as being centered, as in this exercise, is to experience yourself as having a certain presence or "here-ness."

If we get caught up in the push, however, or focus on the person doing the pushing, we place our center outside of ourself. The pusher becomes our center, and when this happens we try to manipulate them or the situation to regain power. This is not genuine power or center. It is one thing to be centered by ourself, and it's an entirely different challenge to be centered while in relationship. If we begin to genuinely experience our own center, we can then receive a push as a gift to help us strengthen and grow. Center is a working alternative to pushing back or being pushed over.

Try this exercise to develop the ability to move from center. First center yourself. Now place both hands, one on top of the other, at your *hara* (Figure 5). Feel or imagine a warmth in this area, and a sense of weight and substance. Now begin to move this center forward without moving your feet. Stay relaxed, with the back leg straight, and allow the front leg to bend and take the weight of the torso. When you've shifted your center as far forward as is comfortable, begin to shift it back. Allow the back leg to bend and take the weight of the torso. Do this a number of times until you feel that your center of movement is located at the point in your lower abdomen.

Next, when your center is shifted as far forward as possible, take a step forward. As you begin to move forward from center, it is important to continue keeping your attention in the area below the belly button. As you bring your back foot forward to step, continue to feel or imagine that the movement originates from this center. As you become more comfortable with this movement, allow your arms to swing naturally and your body to be relaxed. Shift your attention to the motion that is originating from *hara*.

As was mentioned before, center is a state or attitude as well as a specific posture or way of acting. It is a state where we come into relationship with our bodily self in a way that is balanced and present. Sweeping through our bodily dimensions with the attention, to feel an overall balance, is the first step in touching the state of center. We line up our structure in order to touch that balance within. Being in a balanced form opens the opportunity to feel ourself, and the dimension of feeling is directly related to center. If we can feel ourself—our sensations, temperatures, weight, rhythms of excitement, and even pains—we are close to or in the state of center. If we are caught in the net of past events, or are planning the future or wondering if we're doing the right thing, then we are not using ourself as center.

Once we begin to relate to the felt, tangible experience of center, we can then use it as a doorway for departure into the realms of intuition, perception, and expression. Center is both an actual physical experience and a working metaphor that can be applied in our daily life. One can be centered in a physical confrontation, in handling important business issues, in working with interpersonal conflicts, or in practicing a spiritual discipline. Centering is not an end in itself but a self-connection that we can carry into our dialogue with others, our work, and the deeper aspects of who we are.

Pitfall

Center is a place of power. As with any power there are certain pitfalls that should be avoided. When a person begins to develop a center, there can be the tendency to make center a stiff way of being. The trap is in making the means an end in itself. Always working to be centered, we form an attitude that says something like, "I am a centered person, therefore these transitions won't affect me." In a certain sense, an individual who does have a strongly developed center can appear unaffected by outside forces, but there can be a loss of openness and flexibility.

Overemphasis on center creates a rigid, one-dimensional quality. You see it a lot in the martial arts and meditative communities, where so much emphasis on *hara*, being calm, or tan tien (Chinese for "center") makes people strong but distant. The feeling is that there is only center and that it has little relationship to anything but itself. Relating to center in this fashion increases narcissism. If we are in this state, we say, "I am the center of myself and the universe. All things revolve around me." What we forget is that even though center is an important and fundamental state, it is only a stage to help us develop and access other parts of ourself.

It is important to remind ourself that the power of center is in assisting us when we feel lost or anxious. If we stop here or at any of the other stages, we lose sight of the larger vision, and we lose our ability to expand and grow.

Ground

Having established a working center, we can now develop our ground. If center is our application of our personal energy source, then ground is our connection to the qualities and capacities of that energy. Ground comes from directing the bodily streamings, feelings, and sensations of the change in a downward flow. Whether this energy is presently being used to squeeze the lower back, to hold the breath, or to recoil from others or extend toward them, we can use it to ground and connect us to our legs and the earth. This means that the energy released during transition can be used as a grounding force.

If we are suddenly overwhelmed with perceptions, insights, or thoughts, we can use the bodily energy that arises from our confusion to ground us. If the insight is "I'm confused," the next step is to feel the confusion in the body. We can then shape this energetic feeling into a downward flow that is in harmony with gravity. This flow downward, out of our thoughts, establishes a bodily ground from which we are able to grow, just as the infant grows from the loving and supportive ground offered by nurturing parents.

By channeling our energetic and bodily experience through our legs and into the earth, we become grounded in the living reality of our situation. This grounding takes us out of our ideas and connects us to the earth and gravity. Grounding makes things tangible, concrete, down-to-earth. If we allow an energetic charge to run freely down our legs and into the earth, we can respond from a grounded sense of who we are, and not from our conditioned tendency.

If we are struck with a rush of energy and then jump into thinking about how to respond, our behavior will be superficial and immature. We all know people who go around spouting great messages but who are not grounded in what they are saying. They don't have their legs on the ground. They can intelligently talk about knowledge and information, but they are not grounded in that knowledge.

There is wisdom in the excitement that moves through us in times of change. We need to experience that wisdom bodily, to let it ground us, and to then act from that ground. You can experience grounding, as you read by feeling your feet solidly on the floor and your seat resting firmly on your chair. When you speak to someone do so from the feeling of sensations and energy in your feet and legs. Speak and listen from the feeling of being rooted, through your legs, to the ground.

The experience of literally establishing ground can be a very powerful one. A couple I know used the principle of grounding to get themselves out of a tight spot while they were vacationing on a Caribbean island. They had wandered into the wrong side of town, when suddenly they found themselves in a dark and lonely spot with three large men walking menacingly toward them. Having had only six months of aikido training, they were hardly prepared and were, of course, quite frightened. Feeling cornered and not knowing what to do, they did what they had learned: they grounded themselves. They stood in the aikido stance we call *hammi*—they relaxed their knees, lowered their center of gravity, and extended energy out their hands. This is the same stance shown in Figure 1 and is the basic form used for grounding.

After the couple assumed this stance and began to establish their ground, the men suddenly stopped about fifty feet from them. As this man and woman continued to maintain their ground, the men began whispering to each other. After a short time, the potential bullies turned and walked away. It seems that simply being grounded, without retreating or aggressively coming forward, was enough to make these three men think twice about who they were getting involved with.

The experience of grounding that comes from bodily training can be translated to almost every avenue of our life—social, intellectual, and spiritual—and is valuable for such things as dealing with conflict or learning a new skill. Working through the body we can grow and evolve out of difficult situations by learning how to ground ourselves.

Legs as Ground

When we fully experience our legs, we become connected to our support system. Grounding ourselves through our legs, to the earth, gives us a sense of security. If we do not truly inhabit our legs, the movement of our pelvis, torso, and arms, in fact all of our actions in the world, are shaky and have little to support them. There are people who have taut, shriveled legs trying to support large muscular upper bodies. They compensate for this lack of ground by gripping with their toes or contracting their diaphragms or squeezing their buttocks. Their legs arc under them and their feet are on the ground, but not with feeling or energy. Because of the lack of energetic connection between their feet and the ground, they create a ground somewhere around their waist. This makes their actions and gestures tentative and unreliable.

It is not uncommon to find the emotional history of these people marked by a pattern of having been forced to find their ground and support long before they were ready. If they were the eldest child, stories are filled with incidents of being pushed prematurely into walking. If they were younger brothers or sisters, they had to try to keep up and match their older siblings. Somewhere along the line, these people missed a sequence of development and lost an organic connection between their legs and the earth. They look strong and capable on top, but on the bottom they are shaky and groping. These people are filled with doubt and seek their ground in others. In working with these people, first it is important to recognize where they have established their ground—the pelvis, the diaphragm, the solar plexus, the throat—and then to work with their musculature, movement, breath, and sound to bring their excitement and attention into their legs.

Try this exercise with a partner (Figure 6). Stand in a very wide stance, with knees bent and back straight. You should have the feeling of a deep squat while still keeping your balance. Now have your partner stand behind you with their hands pressing straight down on your shoulders. The push should be straight down, such that it does not pull you off balance. Now rise into a full standing position, against the pressure from your partner, in a way that uses your legs and feet. The practice is to come upright by using your ground—the energetic experience of the legs and feet connected to the earth—and not by pushing up with the shoulders and neck. Use this exercise to contact and develop the potential for grounding that is in the legs and feet. You can have your partner use more or less pressure as you work with this aspect of grounding.

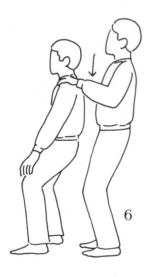

6

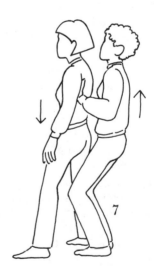

7

Here is another grounding exercise (Figure 7). Stand in a relaxed and centered way. Feel or imagine your energy as a strong flowing current that moves from your belly through your pelvis and legs, deep into the earth. If you start to feel tremblings or streamings in your legs, allow them to join the current that is flowing downward. Now have a friend slowly but firmly try to lift you off the ground by pushing you up from the armpits. Instead of reacting to their push, continue to relate to the flow of your energy into the center of the earth. With some practice, you will feel as rooted as a large tree, and your friend will be unable to lift you.

While practicing the exercise above, add this: extend your fingers and imagine or feel that there are energetic beams coming from them that are being tied to the center of the earth. When your partner slowly but steadily tries to push your arm straight up, it will be as trying to push the earth up (Figure 8).

Pitfall

The trap in overemphasizing ground is that we may become fixed and immoveable. If we are seduced by the power of ground, we often find ourselves so rooted that it is difficult to move. Taking all of our somatic information and channeling it into our ground can make us powerful but also heavy and laborious. When this happens, we lose sight of the potential for being flexible and appropriate while still being grounded. Being grounded, when taken as an end in itself, prevents us from being with others and moving through our obstacles.

8

Entering and Blending

Having established our center and ground, we can now work with the states of entering and blending, in order to work directly with the core of our confusion and change. While the first two stages are an opening and preparation, this stage is marked by our active participation in change itself. At this point we are not only responding to our inner processes—we become involved, through external action, in the situation at hand. We do this by entering into or moving toward our obstacle and then blending or merging with its direction or flow. We decide to trust the intelligence of the somatic information and actively become part of it. In this way, we shape not only ourself but the change itself.

In this stage, because we see a direction open to us, we are faced with a choice. We can go with the movement of "what is," we can resist and go against it, or we can avoid responsibility and deaden ourselves. Entering and blending can take place in the dimension of the literal physical grab, where we experience an attacker's energy pushing in a distinct direction; it can take place in the dimension of a changing relationship, where we clearly see the direction we need to take; or it can take place when we are making a change in career, where we contact new meanings and urges in our life. Whatever the situation, entering and blending can help us work with the flow of energy and events.

Entering

In aikido, we sometimes say that the solution may lie at the heart of the problem, or that the energy of the attack may be its own resolution. There is an aikido movement that epitomizes the quality of facing and moving toward an attack, and it is called *irimi* ("entering"). When an *irimi* technique is called for, we enter directly into the heart of the attack. This entering movement is nonaggressive in the sense that it is done in order to blend with the attack and not to oppose or strike back at it. We move toward the incoming energy, whether it is a physical attack or a verbal tirade, in order to experience it at its essence and then to work with it freshly and creatively.

Entering is not a process of rushing headlong into a problem, but a way of being with ourselves in an open and feeling way. When we begin to turn toward and face our neurosis and unpleasant situations, we are able to work with ourself and our conflicts in a meaningful way. When we no longer run from that which we are afraid of, it is possible to be responsible for our projections of aggression, ignorance, and fear. We also can enter more directly into the core of ourself and our situation.

When we embody an entering movement, we simultaneously become more powerful and more vulnerable. Our step forward says, "I will take the risk of stepping forward and being who I am. I don't know if I'm right or wrong, but I take this risk of moving ahead." In this way, we take on added power and responsibility.

Here's a simple exercise to practice entering (Figure 9). Stand in the *hammi* stance (see Figure 1), centered and grounded. Have a partner walk straight toward you in a committed, resolute fashion. When she gets about two arms' length away, slide directly toward her. Then as she is about to run you over move slightly to the side and turn yourself in the direction that she is moving.

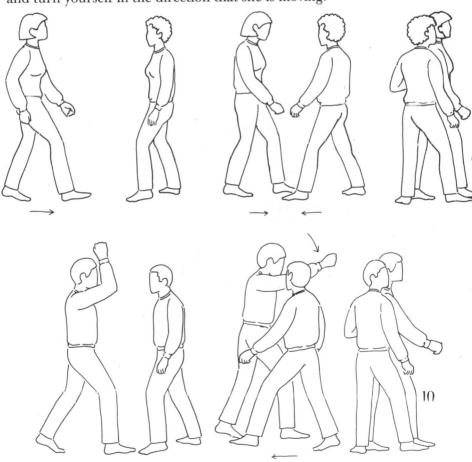

The next step is to have your friend raise her fist as she walks toward you as if to strike you on top of your head (Figure 10). This striking fist can represent any kind of incoming energy—a verbal attack, pressure from your boss, a health crisis, a neurotic attack, or whatever. As your partner comes in, stay centered and grounded and step directly into the attack. At the last minute step aside to avoid being hit and turn in the direction that she is moving. You can have your partner increase the speed and strength of her attack as you feel more skilled.

Blending

In Harper Lee's novel *To Kill A Mockingbird*, Atticus tells his daughter Scout that you never really know a person until you've "walked around in his skin." This is blending. Blending is a merging and joining.

Blending is not acquiescence or weak-hearted submission. It is an active participation that empowers us during change or a crisis. There is a sense of surrender and letting go in blending, but it is not resignation, because it is done from a center and a working ground. Joining with the direction of the energy becomes a form of active nonresistance.

Blending is also a fundamental principle of aikido. When faced with an attack, an aikido practitioner moves in such a way as to blend with the motion and force of the attack. In this way, it becomes possible to use the force of the aggressor to neutralize the attack. By blending with the energy of the attack, we not only know where the attacker is at all times, but we have the possibility, if we are operating from a strong center, to redirect the energy into a nonviolent, spherical motion. By blending with the energy of the attack we are able to see the situation from the attacker's point of view. Once we see and experience the direction of the attacker's energy, blending with it empowers us to direct it and use it.

The following story by Terry Dobson, a fifth-degree black belt in aikido, serves as a dramatic example of the power of blending.*

The train clanked and rattled through the suburbs of Tokyo on a drowsy spring afternoon. Our car was comparatively empty—a few housewives with their kids in tow, some old folks going shopping. I gazed absently at the drab houses and dusty hedgerows.

* Reprinted from the *Lomi School Bulletin*, Summer 1980, pp. 23-24, with permission of the author.

At one station the doors opened, and suddenly the afternoon quiet was shattered by a man bellowing violent, incomprehensible curses. The man staggered into our car. He wore laborer's clothing, and he was big, drunk, and dirty. Screaming, he swung at a woman holding a baby. The blow sent her spinning into the laps of an elderly couple. It was a miracle that the baby was unharmed.

Terrified, the couple jumped up and scrambled toward the other end of the car. The laborer aimed a kick at the retreating back of the old woman but missed as she scuttled to safety. This so enraged the drunk that he grabbed the metal pole in the center of the car and tried to wrench it out of its stanchion. I could see that one of his hands was cut and bleeding. The train lurched ahead, the passengers frozen with fear. I stood up.

I was young then, some twenty years ago, and in pretty good shape. I'd been putting in a solid eight hours of aikido training nearly every day for the past three years. I liked to throw and grapple. I thought I was tough. Trouble was, my martial skill was untested in actual combat. As students of aikido, we were not allowed to fight.

"Aikido," my teacher had said again and again, "is the art of reconciliation. Whoever has the mind to fight has broken his connection with the universe. If you try to dominate people, you are already defeated. We study how to resolve conflict, not how to start it."

I listened to his words. I tried hard. I even went so far as to cross the street to avoid the punks who lounged around train stations. I felt both tough and holy. In my heart, however, I wanted an absolutely legitimate opportunity whereby I might save the innocent by destroying the guilty.

This is it! I said to myself as I got to my feet. People are in danger. If I don't do something fast, somebody will probably get hurt.

Seeing me stand up, the drunk recognized a chance to focus his rage. "Aha!" he roared. "A foreigner! You need a lesson in Japanese manners!"

I held on lightly to the commuter strap overhead and gave him a slow look of disgust and dismissal. I planned to take this turkey apart, but he had to make the first move. I wanted him mad, so I pursed my lips and blew him an insolent kiss.

"All right!" he hollered. "You're gonna get a lesson." He gathered himself for a rush at me.

A split second before he could move, someone shouted, "Hey!" It was earsplitting. I remember the strange joyous, lilting quality of it—as though you and a friend had been searching diligently for something, and he had suddenly stumbled upon it. "Hey!"

I wheeled to my left; the drunk spun to his right. We both stared down at a little old Japanese. He must have been well into his seventies, this tiny gentleman, sitting there immaculate in his kimono. He took no notice of me, but beamed delightedly at the laborer, as though he had the most important, most welcome secret to share.

"C'mere," the old man said in easy vernacular, beckoning to the drunk. "C'mere and talk to me." He waved his hand lightly.

The big man followed, as if on a string. He planted his feet belligerently in front of the old gentleman and roared above the clacking wheels, "Why the hell should I talk to you?" The drunk now had his back to me. If his elbow moved so much as a millimeter, I'd drop him in his socks.

The old man continued to beam at the laborer. "What'cha been drinkin'?" he asked, his eyes sparkling with interest. "I been drinkin' sake," the laborer bellowed back, "and it's none of your business!" Flecks of spittle spattered the old man.

"Oh, that's wonderful," the old man said, "absolutely wonderful! You see, I love sake too. Every night, me and my wife (she's 76 you know), we warm up a little bottle of sake and take it out into the garden, and we sit on an old wooden bench. We watch the sun go down, and we look to see how our persimmon tree is doing. My great-grandfather planted that tree, and we worry about whether it will recover from those ice storms we had last winter. Our tree has done better than I expected, though, especially when you consider the poor quality of the soil. It is gratifying to watch when we take our sake and go out to enjoy the evening—even when it rains!" He looked up at the laborer, eyes twinkling.

As he struggled to follow the old man's conversation, the drunk's face began to soften. His fists slowly unclenched. "Yeah," he said, "I love persimmons too. . . ." His voice trailed off.

"Yes," said the old man smiling, "and I'm sure you have a wonderful wife."

"No," replied the laborer. "My wife died." Very gently, swaying with the motion of the train, the big man began to sob. "I don't got no wife, I don't got no home, I don't got no job. I'm so ashamed of myself." Tears rolled down his cheeks; a spasm of despair rippled through his body.

Now it was my turn. Standing there in my well-scrubbed youth-

ful innocence, my make-this-world-safe-for-democracy righteousness, I suddenly felt dirtier than he was.

Then the train arrived at my stop. As the doors opened, I heard
the old man cluck sympathetically. "My, my," he said, "that is a difficult predicament, indeed. Sit down here and tell me about it."

I turned my head for one last look. The laborer was sprawled
on the seat, his head in the old man's lap. The old man was softly
stroking the filthy, matted hair.

As the train pulled away, I sat down on the bench. What I had
wanted to do with muscle had been accomplished with kind words. I
had just seen aikido tried in combat, and the essence of it was love. I
would have to practice the art with an entirely different spirit. It
would be a long time before I could speak about the resolution of
conflict.

Blending with someone in therapy or education means working with
them where they are and not from a preprogrammed idea, or a
moral idea, about the right or wrong way of being. When we blend
with someone, we see the world from their point of view. Once we
are able to do this, a whole world of possibilities opens up. For one
thing it creates an alternative to simply having winners or losers in
confrontative situations. Blending or going with the energy of the
situation is pivotal in working with "what is" in our life.

Here are a few simple exercises that are useful in developing
the state of blending.

Stand about 30 or 40 feet apart away from your partner, and
then have him begin walking directly toward you. When he is about
three feet from you, step to the side, allowing him to continue his
walk. Then as he passes, begin walking next to him. As you walk
next to your partner, see if you can enter into and blend with his
rhythm, speed, and length of stride. As you continue the exercise
blend as deeply as possible with your partner—breathe like him,
swing your arms the same way, take on the attitude of the walk. Is it
aggressive, timid, relaxed? Try to blend with your partner so thor-
oughly that you feel that you are beginning to wear him as you
would a coat. Begin to feel his walk so deeply that you begin to feel
what it is to actually be this person. Blend so deeply that you can
feel yourself in his skin. This same exercise can be done solo by
blending with walking itself. Give yourself over as totally as possible
to walking.

The next exercise can be done with a partner or by yourself and has three sections. In the first section, have your partner grab your index finger and slowly but firmly bend it backward. This bending pressure will represent a direction of movement, a process in action. In the first section, see how far your finger can be bent while you resist the direction of the bending. When the pain becomes too much, tell your partner to stop. In the second section, take your attention some place very far away—to your place of work, to a memory, to some distant location. Make a note about how far the finger can bend while you "leave" the situation. Most likely it will bend farther than when you were in active resistance. In the third section, actively blend with the direction of the bending finger. In effect, you will be saying, "There is a certain pattern of movement that is going on. I may not like it or even agree with it, but it is happening, so I will blend with it and see what happens if I begin to work with it instead of resisting it." It will soon become evident that by blending with the movement, you feel less pain and the finger is able to bend much farther.

In this next exercise, stand facing your partner with both of you in right *hammi*, that is, with right foot forward (Figure 11). Have your partner point his finger at your chest. This can represent a point of conflict. First feel what it is like to go directly against his energy and intention. Now enter to his right side and blend as totally as possible with his position. Do this not only bodily but also with your attitude. See the world from his point of view. Now that you've entered and blended with his position, feel his weight, his balance, his power, and the commitment of his intention, and blend with them.

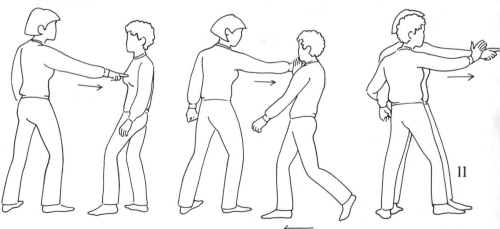

11

Pitfall

Learning how to enter into and blend with the core of our own experience can extend into perceiving the process of others, of organizations, of systems. This is a natural development and not a problem in itself. But if the allurement of this power is such that we are constantly playing "gotcha" or "I see what you're doing," then we have lost our own direction.

Another syndrome of this stage is one that often strikes therapists and teachers. In finding the power to accurately see another, the counselor or therapist will often forget about their own need for growth and introspection. What compounds this is feedback from others about how well we perceive or what great insight we have, or their belief that we must have some kind of magical gift. This kind of attention is often extremely difficult to pass up. We must stay honest with ourselves, and see if we are being seduced into a power game, and then move on to the next stage.

Skillful Actions

We have entered into and blended with the energy of the change, and now we can use the appropriate effort to work with it. We have seen that our transition and confusion has a direction or movement. If we stay aligned to this energy, it is possible to skillfully manage it. There is no need to hurt our grabber or overwork ourselves in dealing with the grab. Because we have a panoramic awareness in this stage, we can make our choices and actions skillful, compassionate, and imaginative.

The stage of skillful action is a deepening into our somatic experience that adds yet another level of vividness and vitality to our lives. The guiding principles of skillful action are positive/extension, receptive/allowing, relaxation, and timing. In this stage, we can develop our own sense of power while still being sensitive to the needs of others. We know how much to extend and how much to receive. Our sense of relaxation and timing is such that we know the moment to act and the moment to do nothing.

This, again, is not simply an idea of how to be or how we "should" be, but a bodily experience that comes from living and acting in the present moment. In other words, our reference point for working skillfully continues to be the body and not cultural or moral precepts. Try the simple exercise of sitting in a chair. Sit with a center and with a ground, and enter and blend with the direction of sitting. Now begin to fine tune and establish a practice of sitting. How can you organize yourself so that sitting is as effortless and full as possible? Can you shape your spine straight and relaxed, with the chest and stomach soft and open? Can you refine your breath so that it becomes a wave, gently massaging the spine? How can you move from sitting to standing in a way that your movements are graceful, centered, grounded, and in harmony with the situation? How can you bring spontaneous gesture and speech into the process of sitting? These questions suggest a way of being that is at the core of this stage of moving through change.

Positive/Extension

Being positive is reaching out, having our energy moving out for contact. It is extending our energy in a positive manner. When we are asked to take a positive stance, most of us usually become aggressive, stiff, and off balance in a forward direction. Emotionally we often misinterpret positive as bullish and ambitious. This is a misinterpretation of being positive and part of the popular narcissism of "I'll do my thing with or without you." But the experience of being positive is not created by erasing someone else's line so your line can look larger. It is the expressing of your own life without dominating or suppressing someone else.

In aikido we call this positive flow of energy "plus *ki*" or "positive *ki*." It is the ability to energetically flow outward without being rigid or frenzied. This self-extending increases our range and reach, whether it is to receive, to push away, or to take. Physically it is exemplified in the golfer, whose energy and attention are both at the handle of the club, where the hands grip, and at the tip, where the head of the club makes contact with the ball. The same is true of someone who holds a paintbrush, a baseball bat, a sword, or a fishing rod. When we extend in this way, we are present in both our center and our ground as we extend out into the environment.

Try this with a partner (Figure 12). First stand in the *hammi* stance, centered and grounded, with the right foot forward. Now put the right arm straight out, elbow slightly bent and shoulder relaxed, with the right hand pointing in the same direction as the right foot. Now feel or imagine that a current of powerful energy is flowing through and out of this arm for a distance of a thousand

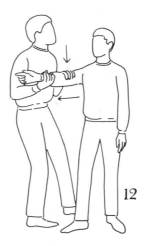

12

miles. Your arm is like a conduit for a limitless and far-reaching energy that effortlessly flows through it. When you start to feel tingling, vibrating, or streaming sensations in your body and arm, continue to relax, and allow these sensations to join the current that is flowing through your arm.

Now ask your partner to put one hand on your bicep and the other hand under your wrist and to slowly but firmly try to bend your arm. Even though he may be stronger, he will most likely find it impossible to bend your arm if your positive flow of energy is steady and relaxed.

The quality that you feel in this arm is that of a positive flow of energy. If practiced enough, this quality can be experienced throughout the entire body. We can then take it into our lives as a way of developing our spirit and making contact with others.

Receptive/Allowing

Receptive is a gentle and sensitive form, but it is not without its positive nature. It has a drawing power that can magnetize and attract. It is the yin force that is often associated with the moon, intuition, yielding, and the Mother. When people misinterpret receptivity, they think being receptive means being wishy-washy, and they usually dig themselves into a hole where their only way out is to become passive-aggressive. They establish a false receptivity by becoming limpid and agreeable, and under pressure usually become aggressive. This is the person who only smiles when angry. Instead of expressing their opinions, these people agree in front of you and later act out their aggression behind your back.

This way of interpreting receptivity usually begins during early childhood. During the process of socialization, parents must necessarily say "no" to the child, but taking away the child's "no" is a mistake. If the child feels that she can only receive and take orders without exercising her own power of "no," which is a basic mode of self-formation, she will become acquiescent and self-denying. She will not only lose the basic experience of receptivity, she will also begin acting out in destructive, passive-aggressive ways.

When working with exercises to cultivate receptivity, it is important to firmly establish ground and center; otherwise receptivity appears to be something noodley and lacking tone. If ground and center are established, receptivity becomes the quality of allowing something to come in without giving up our boundaries or sense of self. There are a number of simple exercises to encourage this.

In this exercise place your hands on your partner's body, bring your attention to the contact of the touch, and be receptive to the communication of the meeting. Place your hand on his stomach while he is standing, and ask him to relax his stomach and diaphragm. Doing this exercise will help you feel the subtle nature and power of receptivity. Releasing the jaw is another way of contacting this quality. Sometimes sitting quietly and being touched by the light of the day or by the sound of chimes, or seeing a piece of art, or even sitting in silence can be a way of contacting a nourishing receptivity.

Try another exercise in receptivity (see Figure 13). First come into the position with the extended arm that was described in the previous section. Then have your partner stand in front of you and

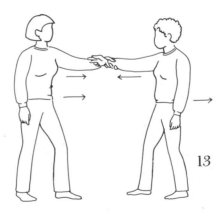

13

grab, from underneath, the wrist of your extended arm. Keep the arm relaxed and the positive energy flowing. This time your partner will push toward you, and you should allow your body to be receptive and receive the push while your arm continues to extend positive energy. In other words allow yourself to be pushed back in relationship to your partner's effort, but keep your arm extended and relaxed. What you feel is the experience of being receptive without being bowled over. As you become comfortable in this exercise, have your partner turn you left and right and push at different speeds. This will fine tune your ability to be receptive while still being centered and grounded.

The T'ai Chi push-hands exercise is a way for two people to study both positive and receptive (Figure 14). Face each other each with the right hand and right foot extended on a diagonal line. Have the backs of your right wrists lightly touch, leaving the hands extended. Then begin moving the hands in a horizontal, circular motion, as if stirring something in a large pot. Each partner takes turns positively directing energy to the other and then receiving the other's energy through the hand and wrist. If your positive extension is too forward, your partner will be able to pull you off your center. If you are overly receptive in the receiving of your partner's energy, your partner will be able to push you off your center. If there is a balance within each partner, and between the partners, the push-hands exercise can help develop the states of positive and receptive.

It seems to be in our nature to have a predilection for the expression of either positive or receptive. It is usually when this

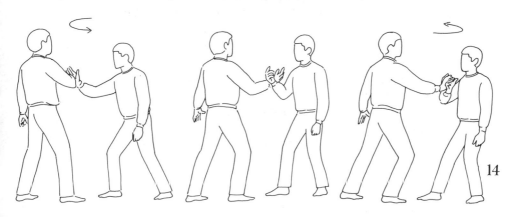

14

predilection becomes an evasion of the other that we are out of balance. Doing exercises and practices associated with these states will usually, after time, bring the insight that the line between being positive and being receptive is very thin indeed, that to be truly receptive we must also be positive, and vice versa. When we come to this understanding, we also draw closer to the experience of relaxation.

Relaxation

Relaxation is as difficult to talk about as it is important. As an athlete, I remember coaches and trainers always saying "Relax," but they were never able to express, experientially, what relaxation was. It is clear, however, that relaxation is fundamental to growth, learning, and health. It is almost impossible to adequately express in words what it is. Nevertheless, the fact is that when we are relaxed we have more energy and we enjoy ourself more.

For most of us, when we say we want to relax we usually mean we want to collapse and not be bothered by anything. But the relaxation that we are referring to in this section is a much more active state. This kind of relaxation is a dynamic calm in our thoughts, feelings, sensations, and actions. It is keeping our spirit, or attention, bright and alive throughout our entire body, while we allow our muscles, tissues, and cells to actively submit to the force of gravity. This notion of relaxation includes the experience of lying or sitting quietly for a few moments and the experience of relaxation as an ongoing, moment-by-moment path.

We may expand our understanding of relaxation by looking at some studies done with infants. Dr. Peter Wolff, of Children's Hospital in Boston, has termed the "quiet alert" state in the infant as one of relaxation.[1] In this state, the infant is bodily relaxed and the eyes are open and appear "bright and shining." The quietly alert infant is able to follow visual and auditory movements while the breathing is regular, rhythmic, and constant. Dr. Wolff states that the child is alert because she wants to be alert and not because she has just awakened. Thus he makes a distinction between being *awake* and being *alert*. The quality and power of our attention when we are alert, in other words, proceeds from a relaxed body. Wolff points out that the child who wishes to be alert, in order to pay attention to an object of interest, first quiets herself down by relaxing her body from crying and disturbance.

[1] Peter H. Wolff, "The Development of Attention in Young Infants," *Annals of New York Academy of Sciences*, New York: 1965, pp. 815–830.

Studies of the nervous system show that the quietly alert state is the optimal state of the reticular formation, a mass of nerve cells and fibers that organizes all activity in the brain, muscles, and vital organs. The reticular formation regulates muscle tone, equilibrium, reflexes, and the muscle readiness we experience in stressful situations. These regulations in turn help determine our qualities of uprightness, strength, grace, efficiency, adaptability, and spontaneous ability to respond. In other words, they direct the flow of consciousness. The quietly alert infant who is relaxed and stimulated to pay attention is most likely to develop a reticular system that maintains strength and relaxation in the muscles, healthy circulation in the organs, and mental growth in the brain.

In the quietly alert state of relaxation, the organ of attention is balanced between sleep and overstimulation, between stress and uninterest, and between emotional reaction and indifference. In the balance between positive and receptive, we are neither hyperactive nor limp and raglike but are alert and interested, and our body is relaxed. We are like the quietly alert newborn.

In aikido practice, relaxation is strongly emphasized and is often the reference point for the different movements of the art. If you try to deal with an attack without being relaxed, you will soon find yourself struggling with the attacker. If you're too stiff, you become brittle and easily breakable. If you're overreceptive, you will be bowled over. In dealing with the grab of an attacker, one's quality of relaxation can help subdue the aggression of the attacker. If we are not relaxed, our panic will only add to an already panic-ridden situation.

In aikido, we practice forms and exercises that increase our ability to relax in a variety of situations, situations in the training hall as well as situations in our daily life. Once we are able to relax with ourself, we are able to execute techniques with precision, force, and compassion. If we are not relaxed, our techniques will be hurried, rough, and colored with fear. To relax is to allow our body to actively participate with gravity while our spirit is upright, alive, and extended. Relaxation can be something we do now and then, or it can be an ongoing practice of working with ourself.

Timing

When the Cambodians began to restructure their culture in the refugee camps, the first two elements that they recreated were dance and music, followed by sports, the Buddhist temples and Christian churches, and finally the schools. Their example underscores the importance of music and dance, which are found in all human cultures, and the underlying principle of rhythm or timing.

There are many stories that establish the ancient alliance between healing and music. Apollo was the god of light, healing, and music, and Asclepius, son of Apollo and god of medicine, prescribed music as an antidote to loss of balance. Music evokes numerous emotional states, and the rhythm or timing of music often resonates with an inner pulse that moves us in unified, coordinated, and well-timed response. This kind of response can be described as being in the right place at the right time.

Timing is present at the moment when we skillfully move out of the way of the aggressor's grab. We are neither behind ourself, nor too far out in front of ourself. Timing in this sense is present when an action is an appropriate response to the present situation, while also being in harmony with an inner rhythm. Timing is not thought out or rehearsed ahead of time, but comes from the instinctive wisdom of the body. It is a knowing that originates from a state deeper and more subtle than logic, reason, or intellect. When we are walking down the street and we skillfully, but unknowingly, jump out of the way of a careless driver, that is timing. When we, for reasons unknown to ourself, suddenly take a new route home and later find out there was a huge accident on our normal route, that is timing. There is no cognitive rationale for this kind of timing; there simply was a response within that moved us at the right time to the right place. These are unexplainable events, but our energetic sense confirms their power and wisdom.

Here is an exercise to work with rhythm and timing. Center and ground yourself while sitting in a chair. Agree that sometime within the next three minutes you will stand. The timing practice is to settle inside yourself so you begin to make contact with that place that says, "Now is the right time to stand." Distinguish between the message from the mental process that may say "You *should* stand now" and the deeper bodily signal. Everyone's signal will be different. It may be an impulse, a sound, a certain feeling of rightness, a quality of movement, a change in vibration. Do the exercise a number of times, and feel what part of yourself tells you it is the appropriate time to act.

Next, stand in a centered and grounded way next to a large pillow. Agree that within the next few minutes or so you will jump over the pillow. Again settle into yourself, and while recognizing the initial urges to react and jump prematurely, wait until you receive the signal within before you respond. The last stage of the exercise is to stand next to a low bench, the task being to jump onto the bench. Moving through this entire exercise from standing to pillow to bench, you will feel an increasing amount of pressure or responsibility. As you increase the pressure, feel how this affects your timing cue. Pay particular attention to the balance between going so deeply inside that you lose the moment of response and being too quick on the draw and moving too soon. Listen to your internal voice in such a way that the distance between the signal and the action becomes very small. This is an additional refinement of the relationship between urge and action.

Some of us are in touch with our needs and urges but seem to be completely in the dark about how to respond to them. We get the message, but instead of acting we analyze it to death. Others of us are constantly in action but are out of touch with the impulse that triggers our actions. To bring urge and action together by tapping our internal timing and rhythm is to integrate our relationship to the inner and outer worlds.

Pitfalls

People who specialize in skillful action often begin to report such phenomena as the ability to see and read auras and energy fields, or they suddenly have access to psychic potential or extraordinary healing abilities. Practitioners of dance, theatre, and martial arts develop an ability to predict an opponent's move before it is made and can then respond with a spontaneous and unique counter. These are meaningful and rich experiences, but they can also become small, isolated pools tucked away from the main current of our life. If we get overly involved in these powers we acquire a certain authority but we may also be sidetracked before completing our transition. We may gain a specific power at the sacrifice of a more total integration of who we are.

We don't need to shy away from any of these abilities or, even worse, try to evade them. However, we do need to be aware of the seductiveness of their power and to exercise caution that our ego doesn't identify with them to the extent of puffing ourself out of proportion. It is possible to come into such powers and not become a more complete person. In fact, these powers can interfere with our growth. If they are a result of living our life and following our urges, we should use them to the best of our ability. But if we use them as a way to control and dominate others, or gain a personal reputation, we may restrict our ability to achieve wholeness.

Union

From the stage of skillful action, we now move to the stage of union with our transition. At this stage we have embodied the transition to such an extent that we are not separate from it: we are the change. The transition is complete, and without hesitation or judgment, we are a channel for the energy that is moving through us. Standing firmly on our feet there is delight and awe in the experience of union with ourself and with the situation.

Union is fundamentally different from the other stages in that it is more a state of being than a conscious act. Trying to describe this experience is difficult in that we do not necessarily have self-awareness while we are in the state. It is an experience where there is awareness, but it is not self-conscious. It is as if we are a transmitter or channel for an energy that touches both our core and the world with which we interact.

If we separate from the state in order to reflect on ourself, to report on our actions, or to write a mental postcard saying, "Gee, I'm doing great," then we are looking at the state instead of being in it. In other words, it is not a time to be aware of ourself or evaluate our actions. It is a time to fully surrender to and stay in the middle of the energetic current that is moving through us. It is a time to fully be our expression. If it is love we are expressing, then we are the embodiment of love. If it is grief, then we are the embodiment of grief. If it is reaching out, then our reaching out is without consideration or reserve. We have become the reach, physically, emotionally, intellectually, and spiritually.

Up to this point, our bodily participation in the transition has been to deepen and intensify feeling and perception, and this intensification has created a structure that has expanded to its full potential, like the unfolded segments of the open telescope. Now we need to let go of the structure and be in union with the purpose it serves.

Think of the person who is preparing to compete in a marathon. The months of preparation preceding the race are a structure in which the runner builds endurance, practices different techniques and styles of running, works out a race strategy, learns an appropriate pacing, and so forth. This pre-race training, which is his personal moving through change, builds a bridge that takes the runner to the day of the marathon itself. The qualities and principles of this bridge help the runner move through the space between getting ready for the race and the moment the starting gun goes off. At the time of the race however, the runner must let go of the bridge and concentrate fully on the race. This means that he must be in union with the things he has practiced, because he is now no longer practicing. He now needs to be those things. Having embodied the elements of the bridge, he allows his training to come through as he completely focuses on the running of the race.

There are no principles to discuss in this stage, because the state of union is a culmination of all that we have discussed already. However, we will later discuss practice, even though we are not practicing anything here or trying for something. We are simply allowing ourselves to be moved by what we have set in motion. We are channeling an energy that is the completion and totality of who we are at that moment.

Teachers who do not understand this state will often interrupt a child whose work or play has brought them into the experience of union. Inadvertently, these teachers, or we as parents, will intervene to ask a question or check to see if the child's experience is one that we approve of or not. This only breaks the child's quality of concentration. What we need to remember is that in this place the child or student is acting without hesitation or judgment. The student is learning not because she is studying something or trying to integrate the material but because she is totally in union with the material itself. She is at one with what she is doing, and this creates union with the material being studied. At this point the student is the laboratory, the material being studied, and the result.

The state of union also serves to remind us of our spiritual nature by invoking the feelings of awe, wonder, delight, meaning, and purpose. It confirms our urges and desires for that which is larger and more universal than our ego routines of struggle, manipulation, and strategizing for power. Union is not simply an idea about our spiritual nature but an embodied experience that manifests itself as a directness and openness in our everyday life. When we are in a state of union, our cells, actions, and thoughts work in rhythm with a higher order and intention.

Because we continue to work from the embodied state, we do not float off with our spiritual inspiration. We can manifest the qualities of the spirit in the here and now of the body. There is no ritualized way to be, there is no need to withdraw from the world, there is no need to wear special robes or to act in any special way. When we are involved with what we are doing, we naturally become a gateway for our more universal natures. Our practice is to simply stay open and allow our excitement to move through us while we interact with the world.

At this level, learning is deeper and more integrative than cognitive memorization or intellectual understanding. This kind of knowing happens from the inside out. All of the stages and states that have been discussed so far have created the condition for this wholeness to occur. But this state of union happens at its own pace and cannot really be controlled. Up to this point, we have given everything we can, both in quality and quantity; now it is a matter of surrendering to the energy that comes through us.

A musician, who I will call Arthur, went through a transformation in his work that exemplifies the state of union and its inherent potentials and problems.

Arthur

Arthur is a virtuoso musician whose career was just beginning to take off when I met him. He had played with many bands and many musicians, and he had just then begun to gain a reputation in his own right. As he said, "People are now paying to see me. They're not paying to see somebody I play with, but they're coming for me and my music." This, of course, was what he had been working toward. There was also a price to pay for this newly acquired success. Now that the spotlight was his, Arthur had become tense and fearful. He lived, in fact, in an almost ongoing state of anxiety, which peaked when it came time to perform. Arthur's inability to deal with his anxiety pushed him to drugs and increasing doubt about himself.

In Arthur's initial work, he established a ground and a center from which he could experience the capacity and qualities of his excitement. He first learned to identify the muscular attitude of his conditioned tendency and then to use the excitement of the neurosis to reshape himself with more flexibility and ground. In some sessions, we would work directly on Arthur's body and his breath; other times, he would practice centering, grounding, blending and relaxation exercises. He also learned the process of how to move from his anxiety to a place of balance and awareness. Because his livelihood depended on it, and because he was committed, Arthur was a will-

ing student who took the exercises into his daily life. After a few
months, his overall sense of anxiety diminished, and he began to
face his performances and rehearsals without the use of drugs.

But as Arthur began to perform free of drugs and free from
the paralyzing grip of his anxiety, he noticed something missing in
his playing. His technique was flawless, but it lacked a certain spirit
that had always been unique to his style. Something was gone. He
was stiff and too held in. In using the states of grounding, centering,
and blending as a glue for his excitement, he had overworked them,
and that had made him stiff and rigid. True, he was calmer, but the
way he shaped his calmness made his playing too predictable. He
played textbook-perfect violin and saxophone, but it didn't thrill.
Even though Arthur felt less abused by his anxiety, he also felt less
excitement. "There's no delight," he said.

What Arthur was doing was jamming up the opening to his creative unconscious with his effort and will. The stage of union could
never really manifest, because Arthur was too busy working on himself and keeping himself on track. Because of all of this busyness,
his spirit never had the opportunity to come through, and his play
lacked zest and spontaneity. Instead of letting go on stage and trusting the body of knowledge that he had been practicing, he continued to practice, and that was the demise of his artistic expression.

With this in mind, he then experimented with letting go of his
conscious effort while performing. The difficulty in his process was
one that many of us have in many different situations. He would enter into a state of union with his music, and then he would suddenly
pop out of this state with a phrase like, "Gee, look what I'm doing,"
or "Am I doing it?", or "This is too intense; I don't know if I should
be here or not." Sometimes he would say these words, and sometimes this was simply the expression of his attention and attitude.
Every time he did this, he took himself out of the state of musical
union.

When he understood what was happening, Arthur decided to
lay aside his practicing and questioning until after the performance.
While he was in the performance, he didn't have to be anything
else; he only had to be. After his sessions, we would evaluate and
critique, but while he was on stage he only had to concentrate on his
music and his playing. Since he had a structured time for feedback,
Arthur felt more room to open and allow the spirit of his music to
flow through him while performing.

Arthur used a simple exercise to experiment with his ability to stay in the state of musical union while at the same time being grounded and centered with his performance anxiety. He would stand in a position that represented the Arthur who was anxious and afraid and then would take the time to muscularly experience the shape, attitude, and quality of excitement of that character. Next he would take a step backward and assume the character of the Arthur who identified with the process of his excitement and not the content. This was the Arthur who could feel instead of worry and the Arthur who could utilize the skills of center, ground, relaxation, and so forth. He would then take the time to experience the qualities of that Arthur. Then he would take a third step back and take the position of the Arthur who was identified with a complete state of being. This was not the anxious Arthur or the Arthur practicing being centered, but the Arthur who was at one with his experience.

In each of the steps, he would consider these questions: What is the quality of my energy in this shape? What is in the foreground of my awareness? What is predominant in my perception?

He would then go through the same sequence while playing his violin. He was to play first like the anxiety-ridden Arthur. Then he was to take a step back and play like the Arthur who was centered, grounded, blending with the situation, and appropriately positive or receptive. Then he was to take another step back and play like the Arthur who was neither identified with anxiety nor practicing the principles of embodiment. When he reached the third step, he played with an abandon and passion that honored his many years of experience.

Playing music in the structure of the three Arthurs (the anxious Arthur, the embodied Arthur, the Arthur in union) over and over again brought him into contact with where and how he was using his attention and his energy. Seeing his performance as a metaphor for life, he was also able to apply this understanding to the way he lived his life. Experiencing how he identified with these different states of being, with his body as a reference point, he also experienced how he could choose to move his identity from state to state. A year after these sessions, Arthur said that the work finally felt integrated. "I'm not only successful," he said, "but I'm also enjoying myself."

Arthur's experience is a reminder that we can overprepare ourself, that ultimately life is to be lived and not practiced. In order for our creativity to come to full potential, we must allow our unconscious to be fully open and available. This, of course, means facing both the darkness and the light within ourselves. At some point in our transitions, we simply need to trust our intentions and the energy that gives birth to all life.

Paradoxically, this is the appropriate time to talk about having a discipline. I use the word paradoxical because the stage of union implies a time when we are not practicing; yet the ability to be in this state, to a large extent, comes from having a personal discipline. In fact, union is a result of having a personal discipline. The following paragraphs will hopefully clarify how having a discipline relates to the stage of union.

Discipline

Adaptation to change has been the way that the human species has developed and grown strong. Another way we can continue our evolution is by taking an honest and penetrating look into the nature of our being. One of our main challenges as a species is to inquire into our mind/body relationship and we can do this by cultivating a sense of practice or discipline in our lives. Discipline in this sense does not mean enforcement, but rather how we conduct ourself in the business of living our life. It requires a personal sense of interest, honesty, and openness about who we are. The awakening that comes from this kind of discipline illuminates the tremendous capacity we have for learning and adapting. The body is our vehicle for this journey, and by staying aware of its many voices, we can find a gentleness toward ourself that can also be shared with others

A discipline is a form that we practice every day. We do it not to run away from something or even to get better at something; we do it because it is a way we can be with ourself outside of the hectic pace of everyday living. It is not a substitute for life but a way of reflecting on our essential self in an unhurried way. From this point of view, a practice is not a way of trying to discharge an inner tension so there may be calmness. On the contrary, in some ways a practice is a way to confront that tension and perhaps even to build on it, much like an engineer who will increase the load on an arch so all of its parts will come together more strongly as a unit.

There are many forms that can be used—sitting, chanting, martial arts, movement/dance, walking, yoga—and we will naturally gravitate to one form or another. It is advisable to have a genuine teacher, one who has traveled the road on which we wish to embark.

It is also important to practice with a freshness and openness that encourages our essential nature to emerge from the frantic pace of modern living. If we have an ongoing discipline, we can appreciate and participate in that which is essential and meaningful in a groundless and anxious world. We can use our discipline to connect us with life and not to run from it.

Pitfall

If our longing for or experience of union is not grounded in the lived experience of the body, we begin to evade responsibility, commitment, and intimacy. To separate our bodily life from our spiritual life is a way of artificially separating from life itself. Once we do this, we then separate from others and may end up judging them for the things we dislike in ourself. Using spirituality as a shield for our vulnerability and insecurity keeps the issues of contact and sexuality at arm's length. The experience of spirituality from the bodily and energetic point of view, however, is one of delight and passion. From this view it is not necessary to wear special clothing, act humble, or pretend we don't have a shadow. To integrate our body into our cosmological yearnings is to allow the ocean of excitement to shape and channel our actions in the world.

In this stage, we can also fall into the trap of being "blissed out." This happens when we become attached to the experience of union and then try to hold on to it by constantly imitating it. These are the people who cannot be bothered by the mundane things of the world. Floating on a cloud above everyday life, they forget that everyone has to squat and relieve their bowels. They want to jump over the barnyard, to keep their feet clean, instead of walking through it. Just because they have been touched by something spiritual, they feel that they never have to step on earth again. But the path of living in the body is to enact our spiritual values with our feet on the ground.

The skills and forms that have been presented for moving through change are tools to help us work through the obstacles and confusion in our life. Once these obstacles begin to break down, there is the potential for presence, and contact with others and the environment. In the following chapter, we will look at how both presence and contact emerge from the life of the body.

TAKING IT TO OTHERS

PRESENCE AND CONTACT

"All means prove but a blunt instrument if they have not behind them a living spirit."   Albert Einstein

For a few years I had the pleasure and good fortune to study under Dr. Randolph Stone. Besides being an osteopath, chiropractor, and naturopath, Dr. Stone was a great man and a healer of immense power. He developed a large and complex system around his work that he called Polarity Therapy. He was a round and lovable butterball, but he could also be sharp and penetrating, like a rapier cutting swiftly to the heart of things. He had an endless supply of information and techniques that he generously shared with whomever was open enough to partake of his abundant feast. This was not always easy, as he was a man of prodigious energy; even in his eighties, he seemed tireless in his efforts to help others. I remember how he once alarmed me by quickly swimming past the safety of a rock jetty and into the open sea. By the time I caught up with him he was turning around, and when he reached the shore he began a spontaneous discourse on the energy currents, a favorite topic. I was exhausted and could hardly hear for my panting.

But despite his extensive knowledge and skills, it is his presence and the way he made contact that has stayed with me the most. He treated everyone both differently and the same. He had a genuine and natural sense of compassion that made everyone equal in his eyes, and at the same time he saw everyone for who they were. Dr. Stone put on no airs, but I felt that nearly all of his patients, at least those I saw, were moved by his powerful love and care. I know that I was. He had a presence that touched people, and it was this presence, not technique, that was the basis of his healing. One incident in particular comes to mind when I think about the power of his presence and contact. At the end of a day-long seminar of treating private clients (he always asked for the most hopeless and "incurable" cases), a van pulled up with a young man who two years previously had broken his neck while diving in a shallow pond. It had left him paralyzed from the neck down, and after two years of inactivity, he had grown to over 250 pounds. He was hauled out of the van on a huge sling, and it took four of us to guide his large and unwieldy body down the driveway. Everything about this man seemed gray and deathlike. He wasn't lifeless, but the life that came out of him was bitter and hard. He saw nothing worth living for and he was terribly angry. I recoiled from him, and I saw that everyone else did too. While we were adjusting him on the table, we all seemed to lean away, casting downward glances until the floor was cluttered with guilt and embarrassment.

Finally Dr. Stone came in from the other room, softly humming a tune as he often did. When he came to the table he placed his large hands on this man, and said to no one in particular, "Well, what do we have here?" I nearly fell over. His relaxation and presence were so different from those of everyone else in the room, he could have been from a different planet. But the fact was that he was actually more on the planet than all of us. Standing next to this huge wounded man, with his hands resting on the man's chest, Dr. Stone gazed intently into his angry eyes. He saw the pain and negativity, but he didn't remain there as the rest of us had. It was as if he was looking past the bitterness and into the part where there was still light and inspiration. It was a very small part, so small that everyone but Dr. Stone refused to go there. It was with that tiny speck of life that Dr. Stone began to communicate. It was as if he were fanning that small spark of life with an unspoken but gigantic "yes." Some minutes went by, and then with an air of sudden finality, he broke the silence. "We have to move the energy currents," and his hands made a large sweeping motion from the ceiling to the floor.

For the next hour, he set about doing his manipulations and instructing the rest of us in various complementary pressure points. There we were, moving busily like worker bees tending the queen bee. But at the core of all of this activity was Dr. Stone's steady and life-giving presence. Everything he did, his touch, his gaze, his movements, his words, all communicated a gigantic "yes" to life. Meanwhile, the rest of us continued to scurry around doing this or that, following his instructions. We, too, were being touched by the energy generated in the room.

As Dr. Stone continued to communicate this unwavering "yes," his young patient, slowly and at first imperceptibly, began to go through a change. There was a softening about him, and he began to respond to Dr. Stone's gaze and encouragement. I don't know what this man thought or felt as he looked into Dr. Stone's soft putty face and fierce eyes, but he had the appearance of a baby looking into the face of its mother. He had connected with something in Dr. Stone that nurtured him. Then out of nowhere Dr. Stone's booming voice said, "Lift your arms." The rest of us stopped. Dr. Stone, who never changed his focus, encouraged us to keep going. Then again, "Lift your arms." The air in the room was electric. The "yes" in all of us seemed to merge together into one positive affirmation of life.

Well, that man moved his fingers, his hand, and then he moved his arm a little. I realized that I had been holding my breath, and we all looked at each other in wonderment. Then both matter-of-factly and triumphantly, Dr. Stone said, "You have to move the energy currents. You have to go past the symptoms and to the core of things." His large hands again made the familiar sweeping motion from top to bottom.

My scientist friends always shake their heads at this story, but I was there, along with a few others, and we saw it happen. I have always felt tremendously privileged to have stood witness to something so profound, so simple, and so life giving. What happened in that room confirmed something for me that I had known for a long time but never really acknowledged on the conscious level, that it is the quality of our presence and contact, much more than any method or system, that makes the impossible possible. When I think about all of the people who have really touched me and made a difference in my life, they are those who have done so with their presence. These people who have made a deep and lasting impression in my life—all the way from a third-grade teacher to a platoon sergeant in the Marine Corps, my grandmother, a meditation teacher, an aikido sensei, a therapist—have done so by allowing their spirit, the truth of who they are, to reach out and touch my spirit. After I recognized and acknowledged the power of presence that day with Dr. Stone, it became a cornerstone of my work, my life, and what is taught at Lomi School and Tamalpais Aikido Institute.

The difficulty of defining contact and presence must be acknowledged before we continue. We can experience them, we can feel them in others, and we can be moved by them, but because of their preverbal nature, they are almost impossible to put into words. Presence and contact should be the foundation of the healing and educational professions, yet outside the experience itself, we have no language to describe them. The power of presence and contact is in the experience, and it cannot be nailed down to a "this" or a "that." Their magnetism is that they cleave straight to the heart, because they are the language of the heart. Making contact from an embodied presence communicates the essence of living things. At its most profound, it is the voice and expression of the human spirit. Writing about contact and presence, then, is trying to put into words what is basically a nonverbal experience. In order to understand these elements of bodily wisdom, we need to free ourself from logic and consecutive thinking and to listen with our body and an open heart.

There is a healing power in contact. A deeply felt energetic presence has the power to bring together that which is fragmented, to create balance and clarity from chaos. This is so because genuine contact brings to light that which is fundamentally good and uplifting about the human spirit. The inspiration that follows makes it possible to have a greater appreciation for our life and the life that is around us. Without the spirit of presence and contact, our actions are flat and mechanical. It's not that techniques are unimportant, but they are effective only to the degree to which they bring us in touch with and channel the life energy that informs, heals, and empowers.

Dr. Stone was overflowing with techniques and theories, but his richness came from the presence he brought to a situation. For decades he traveled around the world visiting and researching any healer or system he thought worthwhile. But all of this information was not what made him effective as a teacher and healer, and he was the first to admit it. He would often say that what he did was very

simple. "You have to move the energy currents. You have to go beneath the problem, under the symptom, to get at the cause of
things," he would say, his large hands smoothing and shaping the air
in front of him as he spoke. Sometimes when he did this in front of
a medical-school audience, the Ph.D. in me, and the M.D. in my
friend and colleague Robert Hall, would shrink and turn red. But
deep down we always knew that what he said was true, and living it
has always been what we have aspired to.

When asked how to do this Dr. Stone would say, "You have to
feel the other person inside of you. You have to feel their health and
their sickness inside of you, and then you understand what to do
and you just do it. This comes from the work you do with yourself."
And this was what he did. He would inevitably go to the pivotal issue in a person, where there was the most life, and would communicate directly to that place. Sometimes he would communicate a
tremendous amount of love and care that would virtually melt resistance and negativity. On other occasions he would be sharp and cutting, like the time he told someone, "There's nothing wrong with
you, you're just full of hot air. Get off the table." Many people in the
room looked down and turned red when he said that, but we all
knew that what he said was true. He also said it in such a way that it
turned the person's life around. But it wasn't the words that held the
power. It was the way he said them, and the light and life that came
from his bodily presence when he said them.

So despite his vast knowledge and learning, it was really how
Dr. Stone brought himself to each situation that inspired life and
understanding. In all of the years that I worked with him, I don't
think I saw him use more than ten or twelve techniques. He could
demonstrate and teach an endless amount of technique, but when
he actually worked with people, his spirit simply connected with the
spirit of his client. The few techniques he did use seemed almost in-
consequential.

To understand what Dr. Stone meant when he said "to feel the
person inside of you" and "you have to understand their health and
sickness inside you," we must realize that the ability to perceive, connect with, and assist someone else is directly related to the depth of
connection we have with ourself. Dr. Stone himself had a meditation
practice, and he always had a very real sense of investigation about
the nature of life. Once when asked how he learned all he did, he
replied with a smile on his face, "I sit up late at night."

A way to develop an embodied presence is to have a practice

that in some way includes the body—sitting meditation, martial arts, movement, working with the breath, yoga, walking, dance. Though practicing these different techniques moves us toward a precision and clarity, ultimately we must practice them as a way of contacting this thing we call presence. The technique is a doorway to connect with the energy of presence and then to make contact from this presence. When Dr. Stone was pleased with one of his students, he never said they were doing that technique correctly. He would say, "You will be good at this work. You are developing nicely." Mitsugi Saotome Sensei, an aikido teacher, reminds his students, "We are not practicing *ikkyo* (number one technique), we are practicing *aikido* (the way of harmonizing oneself with the universe)."

Those people who studied with O'Sensei, the founder of aikido, say that it is the energetic presence of the man that has remained with them, more than any specific way of executing a technique. In his later years O'Sensei rarely, if ever, taught technique. It was his students, after seeing a pattern in his movements, who began to label and categorize his various techniques. O'Sensei spoke of the principles and then taught them by embodying them.

If we continue our own practice, we are able to develop in our life, and this keeps us honest and more able to genuinely communicate with others. If through our practice we become less critical of ourself, we will become less critical of others. If we see ourself more clearly, we will be able to see others more clearly. If we can heal ourself, we can heal others. Anybody can talk a good game, but the authenticity of our words and actions comes from a presence that is developed through a practice of discipline.

When our words, perceptions and actions are born out of a living embodied presence, there is a genuineness that inspires and empowers our life. Presence becomes the basic ground or context in which the communication of information occurs. It is the energetic channel from which knowledge emerges and is communicated. An embodied presence is what exists when our entire body is in a state of attention, and it is from there that authentic contact comes forth. Without presence, contact is one-dimensional. It is like telling about something you've heard about, as compared to telling about a first-hand experience.

How strange it seems that, despite its power to heal and inspire, contact plays such a small part in our education and healing professions, to say nothing of our everyday life. Somewhere along the line, the emphasis on getting ahead, accumulating material goods, and climbing to the top of the heap has severed us from the importance of quality human contact. The goal of collecting enough techniques and theories to go out and get a job overrides the underlying importance of presence and contact as the ground from which technique becomes effective.

Contact can take many forms, but the form itself does not guarantee that genuine, spirit-to-spirit contact will be made. A handshake between two strangers can have the power to initiate a lifetime relationship, while two people can spend the night together and make no contact whatsoever. Just because our feet and legs are on the ground does not mean that we are grounded. We establish our contact with ground by allowing our energetic presence to move as a living charge through our legs and feet into the ground. We make contact visually by allowing our presence to move as excitement through our eyes into the environment, not by just looking at somebody. Unexpectedly, but often with great reward, we can find contact in conflict and aggression. As Fritz Perls said, "Contact is the appreciation of differences." Contact can take almost any form as long as we bring an energetic presence to the form.

Contact is how we are with somebody or something. Presence, which is our embodied awareness, is the mother of contact. Contact is the process of transmitting meaningful information through language, touch, emotions, nonverbal gestures, and energy fields, and it originates in our living presence. As our living presence is active and dynamic, so is our contact. Contact offers the possibility of relating to ourself, others, and our daily situations on a moment-to-moment basis. This notion of contact includes our spectrum of awareness.

If technique becomes our goal, this will shield us from the possibility of a deeper connection. I have seen this over and over again in aikido, where someone may be performing a technique letter-perfect, but because the spirit of the event is missing there is no real relationship between technique and partner. When this happens the partner looks like he is being mauled and dragged around the mat. The same thing can happen in bodywork, where the practitioner can have their hands in the right place and be doing the proper technique without really touching the person living in the body. Or it can happen in therapy where the therapist does all of his relating through the style of his system. He may be doing the "right" thing, but his way of relating is flat, overstylized, and unconnected to the person he is working with.

When we make contact, we are able to connect with the spirit of living things. Contact with life can be experienced as a texture, a tone, a mood, a sense, or a feeling, and it is the emerging of presence. Sometimes this quality is very tangible, and at other times it may only be a sense of something. With training in the perceptive and intuitive aspects of the body, we can "read" or sense qualities of presence and contact. This type of perception is like that of the experienced sailor who can "read" the conditions of the sea. There is nothing particularly mystical or magical about what he can see and sense; it is simply a matter of experience. In the same way, if we allow ourself to experience and be touched by life, we can "read" qualities of energy, presence, and contact. Through certain practices, especially in the movement and contemplative arts, this type of perception can be developed so that sensing qualities of energy becomes second nature.

We can feel a probing, cautious quality about some people's contact that says, "I want to go slow and feel if this is safe." With others, there is a radiance that gushes over in its yearning to make contact. When these radiant people are out of touch with their energy, they will often say, "I am giving, available, and open—why does no one respond to me?" They are unable to feel that they don't allow the space for someone to come forward. Another person may ooze a sticky, syrupy quality of energy that is seductive. These people have a carnivorous view of contact that tells them they will be somebody if they can ingest someone else. Other people simply beam and delight us with the lightness and humor that they bring to life. Yet another type exudes a stillness and weight that evokes the image of a center pole, a quiet depth whose level of contact is deeply caring.

Contact in this sense of perceiving and connecting is fundamental to the process of learning. It allows a teacher to see the most appropriate way to approach a student, and it builds a bridge of trust that helps the student learn. It can tell a personnel director something about a job applicant that is not on the resumé. It can help a physician work with a child who is afraid of doctors. It can tell a police officer the best way to defuse a potentially dangerous confrontation. It can inform a parent about the needs of a child who is reluctant or shy in talking about personal matters. To contact the rhythm of someone's excitement is to connect with the deepest and most essential part of them, and this connection creates the conditions for further learning and communication to occur. If we engage a person and their excitement in the learning process, instead of trying to hammer in information, learning can be satisfying in the moment as well as applicable to other areas of life.

Learning to ski last winter, I took a lesson from an accomplished skier and certified instructor. He initially amazed me, as his instructions were similar to the ones I use with my students. He spoke of the importance of relaxation, going with the contours of the slopes, and trusting my body to feel weight, balance, and flexibility. His images were creative and useful. I was inspired and immediately put to use what he was telling me. But after a point, I got stuck. The instructor came over, reeled off his terrific aphorisms, and I again tried to put them to use. But there was no progress. Something was missing.

I realized that he wasn't making contact with me. He wasn't seeing me and what I needed to learn in order to move ahead. His wonderful information lacked a connecting bridge to the more essential part of me. I was left with great tips but with no real ground to learn and to develop. If he had been able to make qualitative contact with me, he could have communicated what I needed to know to inspire me to move forward and improve. As it was, the information was like that on a mimeographed handout. He was simply repeating what he said to everyone, without shaping his material in a way that was meaningful to my learning. When I didn't improve, he became frustrated and increased his outflow of "knowledge" instead of seeing what would be the appropriate thing for me. Perhaps if he had tuned in, he might have brought forth the suggestion to turn my hip a little this way, or lean slightly that way, or even work with the energy of my emerging frustration.

This event brought home that no matter how "new age," enlightened, or philosophically correct an idea, without presence and contact they remain only ideas. Having good ideas without being able to embody and effectively communicate them is like spitting in the wind. Presence and quality contact are the things that make the difference between someone who delivers information and someone who is an inspiring teacher. A quality teacher is someone who can transmit experience and the joy of learning.

Contact is a process that is dynamic, changing, and rhythmic, and the more that contact emerges from an embodied presence, the more powerful and effective it will be. In this process the energetic exchange of information can take place within ourself, between ourself and someone else, or between ourself and the current situation in our life.

Establishing contact with ourself naturally creates the foundation for purposeful contact with others and the environment. We must first learn how to be with ourself before we can truly be with others. Connecting in a responsible way with our excitement cultivates a basic ground from which to mobilize and extend out. We learn that the ways we contact ourself—gently, directly, lovingly, incisively—are also the ways we contact those outside of us. Understanding how we contact ourself helps us to take responsibility for our projections and fantasies.

Contact with others is the natural outgrowth of the connection we have made with ourself. When we are connected with ourself, our excitement automatically begins to flow outward, and we weave the fabric of our lives with the streamings and pulsations of those around us. In contact with others, we enact the ancient excitatory process of forming families, tribes, and communities. Having connected with our own energetic vision, we are able to qualitatively contact those around us.

Contact with the conditions in which the events of life occur offers a panoramic view of our world situation. We see how we affect the environment and how the environment, in turn, shapes us. We experience that everything is in a state of change, that some things are in our dominion and others are unquestionably out of our control. Coming in contact with the conditions of life exposes our vulnerability. This is often painful, and it also shows us the limits of our personal power. But integrating and accepting these limits often gives birth to the awareness of a power much greater than that of personal ego. This inspires us toward openness and acceptance in our life.

Contacting the nature of our situation, which is the situation of life, can bring us to the universal insights of love, service, impermanence, and wisdom. It calls forth genuine yearnings that can only be called religious, in the deepest sense of the word. It invokes awe at the immensity of life and appreciation for our place in it.

Children are testimonies to the power and value of presence and contact. Almost all children, whether they are healthy, emotionally disturbed, juvenile delinquents, or have severe learning disabilities, are clearly more interested in and affected by the qualities of presence and contact than by anything else. When you are present they respond to you. When you leave, they too will leave. If you are beating around the bush, they know it. Because of their sensitivity, working with them is a razor's edge. If you veer even a fraction of an inch, everyone falls over the side. This instant feedback is infuriating, but it is challenging in the presence and contact that it offers.

The urge for contact in children is as great as their resistance to it. This resistance simply says how much they want it, how much we all want it. Children will disguise their need for contact in predictable ways. When they start to argue, they are often only requesting contact. When they fight, they show their inability to handle intimacy, or their frustration with it. If they run off, they are most likely afraid of again being denied the contact they long for. Yet, when they finally allow themselves to connect directly with another person, they soak it up like a sponge. Their eyes shine with warmth and love, and it feels like being at a huge banquet. A powerful comment about contact is the report that almost *all* emotionally disturbed children have had a minimum of, if any, genuine contact in their lives. It is also clear that what has been most instrumental in these children's healing and growth has been meaningful contact.

For about two years, I worked with an emotionally disturbed boy I will call Marvin. Though he kept himself distant from me, I grew fond of Marvin, and I think he grew fond of me. He rarely said anything, but sometimes he would stand next to me or ask me a question in a way that told me he wanted to get nearer but didn't know how or wasn't quite ready. On my end, I saw myself in him, how I was when I was a boy. He was quick, smart, and facile in his accomplishments, but he was also moody and could erupt in unpredictable ways. If he got too close to somebody or began to succeed too easily, he would start a fight or sabotage his efforts in some defensive way. He was close to his mother, but he hadn't really learned how to trust people. He was also athletic, so I would try to reach him through movement and would play with him and try to make as much physical contact as possible.

Sometimes in our play, when I thought we were becoming closer, he would turn on me and deliver some stinging remark. "Why did you do that?" he would shout. "Can't you tell you're hurting me? You don't care about me—if you did you wouldn't play so rough." His voice would rise to a shriek. Sensitive as he was, he felt my need to contact him and my indirectness about it, and he couldn't tolerate it. He knew I wanted something from him, and he knew I wasn't being straight about it, and he resented the way I used that to control him. So he would strike back in the only way that he knew how, through his words, and he could put venom in them. At the same time, he liked me. And so we went on for over a year this way, both wanting contact, both hating each other's needs, both seeing ourself in the other.

Then one day when we were together, doing nothing in particular, I noticed Marvin looking at me intently. I could see that he wasn't running some number on me, like a stare-down or an I'm-watching-you-when-you-can't-see-me routine, because his body was relaxed, his gaze was soft, and his bodily attitude was open. When he saw that I noticed him, he came over, never taking his gaze from my eyes. Sitting in front of me, he looked more deeply and directly into my eyes than he ever had and simply said, "Your eyes are brown." I was stunned. It was not only what he said but how he said it. In that moment I knew and he knew that his vision had suddenly opened. He was looking out of himself, and he saw something out there: it was me, and there was a felt shared warmth between us. His openness opened me, and his contact brought me into contact. My entire body felt alive, and there was a current of aliveness that passed between us.

A simple enough thing it is, someone noticing the color of your eyes. But when we put our heads straight on our shoulders, look directly out at the world, and make contact, there is an illumination that transcends all of the categories of neurosis, double-bind, and emotional disturbance. Some things changed for Marvin after this episode. In noticing more of everyone else's eye color, he also saw a great deal more of each person, and his play became less quarrelsome. What changed for me was realizing that my effort to contact Marvin and these other emotionally disturbed children mostly got in my way, for genuine contact comes from simply being ourself. Always busy trying to be somebody making something happen only gets in our way.

As strong and as natural an urge that the urge to contact is, we all seem unprepared and naive in responding to it. We all want contact, but the intimacy frightens us. We want to connect somewhere, but we don't know how to begin. The excitement that comes with contact makes us anxious. We wonder if we are doing the right thing. When we are finally in contact, we don't know how to separate, to say, "Thank you, that's enough for now."

Then there are the endless accounts of emotionally and physically abused children, who as adults will carry their scars as suspicion, fear, and violence. They are our testimony to the poverty of a life that is barren of contact. In some families, all that gets touched is the dog and the T.V., and when the T.V. goes off, the family members withdraw or make contact by abusing each other. And since we have never been told how to connect with ourself, we feel lost and rejected when we find ourself alone.

Perhaps it is simply that rejection and abandonment are universal issues, and the fear of them gets played out in the arena of contact. Bodies desire to be around other bodies; people long to be with other people. The manipulations and strategies that accompany our desire to love and be loved make contact an issue in almost everyone's life.

An added factor in our confusion about contact comes from the disembodied view of contact presented by society. We are taught that there are good ways of making contact and bad ways. There are the right people to be with and the others to be avoided. We are taught that contact is unlikely if not impossible in conflict situations, when ironically enough, that is often where it is most rich and useful. Young women are schooled that charm and a fixed smile are the avenues of contact. In the man's world, contact is a hearty slap on the back. The media remind us that contact is achieved if we can get the favored lipstick, cologne, the car, or even the hamburger. Our cultural images reinforce the idea that contact is something that is static—a person, a place, or a thing—which implies that once contact is made, that's it until the next acceptable mode is available. This impoverished attitude doesn't account for our natural sense of curiosity or for our basic urge to explore our surroundings and to discover ourself.

Identifying with static media concepts, we become the audience of housewives who turn on the soaps when the kids leave for school, or the therapist who doesn't know what to do with herself when she's between clients, or the executive who feels impotent when he's away from the boardroom. When we rigidify how and where we make contact, we are also freezing our attention, our meaning in life, and our creativity. If you ask someone what gives their life meaning, the answer will most likely lead to the part of their life that is rich with contact and energy. Likewise, if you ask someone what is wrong in their life, their answer will most likely describe a situation where there is little contact or energy.

Instead of trying to learn contact from how-to manuals or from the way the Joneses next door do it, in the somatic way we use the rhythm of our excitement as a guide. This acknowledges that the how of contact comes from the actual experience of living. We learn to make contact by being with our bodies, following our energy, and trusting our perceptions, not by collecting concepts or trying to live a certain way.

Contact that comes from an embodied living presence is the energetic tide of our reaching out and collecting back in. Like a wave that momentarily distinguishes itself from the ocean, builds, crests, reaches to the shore, and then recedes to again collect itself for another beginning, our contact reflects the connecting pulse of life in its ebb and flow. The ways that we awaken, increase, contain, and discharge our energy are the same as our process of contact. The spectrum and richness of our contact reflects the quality of our life and the way we use our energy. Those who are limited in contact are also limited in the way they live their life. Contact and our energy are inextricably tied together, and when they merge, there is meaning. And to best understand how to be in contact, we need to understand our excitement and its rhythms, which is where we began at the beginning of this book. Thus we complete the cycle.

The fruition of working through the body is to take this knowledge into a social context and into the many conflicts that arise in our life and the world. In the next chapter, we will look at the body's knowledge in respect to working with our aggression and the unprecedented violence that is part of our world.

TAMING AGRESSION:
THE AIKI WAY
OF CONFLICT RESOLUTION

"War is but a spectacular expression of our daily conduct." Krishnamurti

The other day there were two stories in the newspaper that stood out. The first was about an English couple who had been turned down in their application to adopt a foster child. Their work and life for the past fifteen years had been running a home, successfully, for orphaned children. The authorities had denied their request because they feared this couple was "too happy." It would be an "unrealistic environment" in which to raise children, they said. They further hinted that a life with more quarreling and tension would better prepare a child for life in the world, and therefore they rejected the application.

The adjoining story was about the war in El Salvador and carried the headline, "Twenty-One Killed in El Salvador: El Salvador Shrugs it Off." Apparently the government forces had refused to pay ransom or bargain for twenty-one kidnap victims, so the hostages had been executed en masse by the rebel side. The government had "shrugged it off" and ultimately refused even to claim the corpses.

The irony in these stories is painfully obvious, and it had the effect, as the media often does, of momentarily distancing me from the actual tragedy of the two events. But as I reread the stories and saw them as separate shingles hanging on the wall of modern times, advertising our present state of affairs. a disturbing question came to my mind: What do we mean by society and culture when life is being shaped by such aggression and lack of feeling?

Most of us need little reminder that we live in a time of unprecedented violence and aggression. If it doesn't come from the litany of destruction that we are constantly fed by the T.V. and newspapers, it is presented to us as the real thing. Assault, rape, murder, and theft are experiences that no longer describe someone else's life. Most of us have experienced some sort of aggressive intrusion into our lives, or we know someone who has been attacked in one way or another. In many ways the basic condition modern society has come to is one of rape. Whether acted out as sexual assault, exploding a bomb in a train station, invading another country, strip mining, ripping off welfare checks from the elderly, or beating our children and spouses, the theme is always the same: dominating or forcibly taking something from another. How do we stop this acceleration of violence? Where does it even begin?

There are three basic approaches that have emerged for dealing with violence and aggression. They can be called the "out there" approach, social programs, and personal work. The first approach, which seems to gather the most support, is to cluster around the major issues—nuclear war, crime, terrorism, drugs, environmental destruction, urban decay, race and religious strife—and begin to define the enemy as "out there."

Let's take crime as an example. Across the country we hear judges and the courts announcing new legal reforms that will "put away for good" the bad elements, as if our lives would be complete if all of the bad people were swept under the great Constitutional rug. Yet as it is, the courts are backlogged with untried cases, and more are on the way. Then we are told that more and bigger prisons may be the answer, even though over 50 percent of convicted criminals return to prison. This high rate of returning alumni makes additional prisons an unconvincing medicine for crime and violence.

The voice of the "out there" approach is also in the defense department, lobbying for money to implement a "get tough" policy. The belief is that toughness, the Big Stick and the flexed bicep, is the missing ingredient. Is it really toughness that is needed? We can no more deter violence with toughness than we can stop a flu epidemic by beating up everyone with a fever. But we hunger for a culprit. We search for a strategy to beat the *bad guys*. If only we could fix something out there, we keep telling ourselves.

Part of the philosophy of this approach indicts humans as genetically aggressive and warlike by fingering our evolutionary past, or by pointing out the territorial aggressiveness we see in the animal kingdom. But the argument that war is indelibly stamped in our genes is simply another excuse for not looking to ourselves for a solution. Both harmony and aggression are a part of our nature, and we don't necessarily have a predilection for either one or the other. The tendency we have toward peace or violence is learned and cultivated culturally. In a single day, our moods may alternate between compassion and hatred countless times. Aggression, like love, simply is.

Continuing to reduce our responsibility for our personal daily ventilations with such modern terms as "high-pressure situations," "anxiety-producing conditions," "low-blood-sugar effects," and "innocent because of temporary insanity," is a bunch of baloney, and it misses the value of looking at the seeds of violence within ourselves. Blaming our genes or something outside ourself for our aggression takes us away from working with the situation as it is.

The second approach looks to social programs to eradicate the possible causes of violence. These programs work with the categories of unemployment, job training, prison reform, overpopulation, hunger, religious and race discrimination, community development, and so forth. These programs are important and should be supported. Though they are often bogged down in bureaucracy, they keep these issues in the public eye and they are often successful in alleviating suffering.

The third approach is to personally work with our aggression in our daily lives. Instead of making someone else wrong, or fortifying a position that makes us right, we can work with what is most common and closest to all of us: our body, thoughts, feelings, emotions, and actions. In this way, we can experience conflict as something that is not only out there, but here—here in the moment of this reading, here in our families, at our jobs, with the people with whom we have most contact. Conflict, like peace, simply is. When conflict becomes damaging is when we deny it or project it onto others.

Many anthropologists hypothesize that our aggression is historically rooted in the domination of nature, which began as our early ancestors made the transition from hunter/gatherers to farmer/tenders. This was a passage that created the idea of property and subsequently the need to defend property. The bodily way we experience this domination of nature today is in the way we separate ourself from what we feel and sense. Through the influence of our educational system, churches, and media, we have learned to dominate and deny the experience of our bodily life. This initial act of aggression against ourselves is only a short step away from acts of aggression toward the environment and others. By dominating or disassociating from the rushes of excitement we experience bodily, we create a struggle within ourselves that tends to spill out into the other areas of our lives. We are simply not taught how to be personally responsible for the power and wisdom of our bodily life. Because of this failure, society is becoming increasingly oriented toward violence and mechanized behavior. The story of a man called Raphael painfully illustrates this point.

When I met Raphael he was probably in his late thirties, and he worked on the streets with the black and chicano gangs of East Los Angeles. He moved carefully, always aware of what was behind him, and his skin was pulled taut across his face. What he didn't want you to know, he could hide behind a mask of icy indifference. When he trusted you, his eyes became a sunny beach and it was easy to relax in his warmth and openness.

Raphael was respected by both the police and the gangs, which was unique. In an environment where loyalty and pride were the most esteemed values, this was no easy task. Raphael came from the streets, had committed its violences, and had risen above them. Perhaps his real story is how he transformed himself from a cold, merciless predator into a genuine caring human; but the one that I was let in on was about the violence that can happen when we remove ourself from our bodily feelings.

When Raphael told his story, he did so hesitantly, like someone carefully touching an old wound. It was clear right away this wasn't going to be the usual war story, full of pride but vacant of deeper feelings and emotions. Raphael was reopening a darkness that had been sealed many years before. When Raphael spoke, the room was silent, and his memories seemed to break off from his body and fill the room.

It seemed that Raphael's mother, who was only thirteen when she gave birth to him, disciplined him early on never to cry. When he was age five or six, she would hang him up by his thumbs as a punishment for crying. If he would cry over this, she would beat him with an electrical cord and then salt his open wounds. Raphael learned how to squeeze and tighten himself so that nothing would come out.

As Raphael told this story, his words came slowly and were barely above a whisper—strange for a man who lived in a world where macho was only a starting point. As he relived these terrible memories, someone asked him what he felt at those times. Raphael stopped for a moment, and after digging deep into his darkness, he said with an excessive quietness, "I just wanted to get back at my mother." Someone then asked, "But what did you feel?" Raphael tightened his eyes as he lowered himself deeper and deeper into the past. After some time, he opened his eyes and said with surprise, "I didn't feel anything. I left my body. There was nothing to feel." We all knew what he was talking about. Feeling was just too dangerous.

Of course Raphael left his body; it was the only intelligent thing to do. If he hadn't, the physical pain of ligaments torn from the bone and the emotional pain of rejection might have killed him. Leaving his body made Raphael a survivor. But looking deeper, Raphael saw that when he checked out of his body to avoid his pain, he also checked out of his other feelings as well. He said that later in his life, he would become infuriated when he would see other people cry. He even went so far as to beat and stab someone if they started to cry. When as a gang leader he would have someone murdered, he would feel nothing. Raphael remembered that when he first became a father he knew he loved his children, but he couldn't *feel* it. Asked if he had told his children that he loved them, which he obviously did, he replied, "I was afraid that if I did I might cry or they might cry, and I just couldn't stand that."

After Raphael left his body, it was easy to hurt others. Without feeling himself, he couldn't feel someone else. But somewhere along the line, he began to take responsibility for himself, his body, and his feelings, and he regained his status as a human being capable of feeling and caring. He now helps chicano and black kids make the change that he did. But his story remains a dramatic reminder of the cost of dying to our bodily life.

We need to remind ourselves that it is not ideologies that bleed in wars; it is people who bleed for ideologies. It is not politicians that fight wars, but desensitized youth who are sent into battle. It is not religions that suffer in pain; it is individuals who inflict suffering on other individuals under the banner of God and country. Those that continue to place the blame for war and violence on others, and deny personal responsibility, are committing the offense of avoidance. What I am suggesting is that until we identify, accept, and integrate our own feelings of aggression, all of the political and social processes, however sophisticated, will be inadequate in dealing with the human dilemma of life on planet earth.

A friend had an experience that relates directly to this issue. It was at a time when he was a single parent for about five weeks while his wife was away on a business trip. During this period, he grew much closer to his children, and his relationship with his thirteen-year-old daughter particularly became more intimate. One evening they stayed up late talking, and when it came time to go to bed the daughter, as he told it, "looked directly in my eyes and said in both total innocence and with the voice of the eternal woman, 'Papa, can I sleep with you tonight?'" My friend recounted that at that point "a huge wave of energy rushed through my body. I suddenly didn't know who I was or how to respond. There was so much heat in me that I felt like I was on fire. I was both confused and turned on. I then became angry that I was turned on and made so vulnerable. At that moment I understood, in a flash of clarity and insight, why so many fathers begin to distance themselves from their daughters. I understood that a tremendous amount of child abuse and sexual molestation in our society comes from the father's inability to identify and deal with the energy that arises out of his attraction to his daughter. In the moment that I felt 'wrong' about my feelings, I could feel how I wanted to lash out at my daughter."

The taboo against incest is such a strong "no" that most fathers feel that something may be wrong with them when these rushes of energy and attraction arise. Not knowing how to face this charged situation, they project their confusion and anger outward. Not taking responsibility for their own feelings and energetic streamings, they make the daughter wrong for their experience. Misunderstanding and unable to tolerate this level of bodily aliveness, and having no tools for being centered and grounded in the experience, they try to rid themselves of these feelings, emotions, and thoughts by blaming the child. If the child is made wrong, in other words, the parent cannot be wrong. In this way, the father, not wanting to confront what is going on inside of him, usually begins to distance himself from his daughter. In extreme situations, this means abusing the child physically and sexually. Fortunately, my friend had the awareness and courage to feel his aggression without acting on it.

Working through the body, it is possible not only to contact the aggression that is within us but to work with it and transform it. At other places in this book I have touched on how to do this through bodywork, breath, movement, and personal processing. It is now time to talk about aikido, a unique martial art, and how it can function as a way to ritualize our violence and integrate our aggressiveness.

Aikido was founded in the late 1920s by Morihei Uyeshiba, a modern-day Japanese samurai. As a young man, Uyeshiba watched helplessly as a gang of hoodlums beat up his father, and he vowed to undertake whatever training and discipline necessary to avenge his father's beating. This vow produced one of the foremost *budo* ("the way of the warrior") masters in the history of Japan. He became a master of numerous martial arts, including sword, spear, staff, and various schools of jujitsu. But O'Sensei ("Great Master"), as he was referred to by his students, wasn't merely satisfied with physical strength and the perfection of technique. After having defeated all comers and surpassing many of his teachers, he began to challenge the value of winning at the expense of the loser. He raised questions about the rightness of using might to dominate others. These issues led him toward a penetrating inquiry into the true nature of *budo*: Is it enough to simply be a winner over another? Is physical strength and accomplished technique the goal of the warrior's path?

During this period of questioning, O'Sensei was challenged to a duel by a naval officer who was also an expert swordsman. As the officer repeatedly charged O'Sensei, attempting to strike him with his wooden sword, O'Sensei would easily move out of the way of the sword cut. Finally the officer, overwhelmed with fatigue, sat down without ever having touched Uyeshiba.

Uyeshiba walked to a nearby garden and was suddenly overcome by a strange and unexpected feeling. As he later recounted:

I felt that the universe suddenly quaked, and that a golden spirit sprang up from the ground, veiled my body, and changed my body into one of gold. At the same time my mind and body became light. I was able to understand the whispering of the birds, and was clearly aware of the mind of God, the Crea-

tor of this universe. At that moment I was enlightened: the source of budo *is God's love—the spirit of loving protection for all beings. Tears of joy streamed down my cheeks. I understood:* Budo *is not felling the opponent by our force; nor is it a tool to lead the world into destruction with arms. I understood: The training of* budo *is to take God's love, which correctly produces, protects, and cultivates all things in Nature, and assimilate and utilize it in our own mind and body.*[2]

This was the birth of aikido. It would be as if the secretary of defense suddenly declared that from now on the duty of the armed forces of the United States would be to serve, protect, and love all people of the world. Of course many came to see and challenge this new *budo* of "peaceful reconciliation," and most of them remained as dedicated students. In those early days, it is said that O'Sensei's school was full of masters and teachers from other martial arts who were awed by the effortless power of this great man. Now aikido is taught throughout the world.

Aikido means the way of harmony with the spirit of the universe. As a martial art, its aim is to neutralize an attacker's energy instead of trying to hurt them. This is done through an entering into and blending with the attacker's force and then leading it into a spherical motion. What then results is the aggressor being thrown to the ground or held in a neutralizing joint-lock.

Aikido is a powerful martial art as well as an aesthetically beautiful one. During training sessions, one sees a spirited group of men and women moving in natural circular movements as they engage each other in strong physical contact. Partners spend equal time being *uke* (the attacker) and *nage* (the one who deals with the attack). Using the entering and blending movements, the *nage* slips out of the way of a punch, kick, or grab and then guides the *uke* in a circular direction until the person is thrown to the matted surface. After falling, which is an art in itself, the attacker energetically springs to the feet and continues to attack until the roles are reversed. Whether one is *uke* or *nage*, what is at the heart of every movement and technique is the expression of reconciliation and harmony. In the words of the founder:

The secret of aikido is to harmonize ourselves with the movement of the universe itself. He who has gained the secret of aikido has the universe in himself and can say, "I am the universe."

[2] Kisshomaru Uyeshiba, *Aikido* (Tokyo: Hozansha Publishing, 1974), p. 5.

Aiki is not a technique to fight with or defeat the enemy. It is the way to reconcile the world and make human beings one family.[3]

Although the graceful movements of aikido appear dancelike, it is an extremely effective self-defense form. The emphasis on centering, grounding, and the extension of energy, or *ki*, provides aikidoists with the training to defend themselves and others, while skillfully preventing serious injury to the assailant. At its most profound level, aikido develops a sensitivity and facility for avoiding and resolving conflict even before it escalates into physical violence.

Aikido is a creative and appropriate form for teaching us how to resolve conflict in ourselves and in our environment, as well as how to work with our competitive nature. There are three factors that especially encourage this potential.

To begin with, the concept of self-responsibility is an underlying foundation of aikido training. In his memoirs O'Sensei wrote, "The only opponent is within. Aikido is not for correcting others; it is for correcting your own mind." This means that as a beginning aikido student you quickly learn that there is greater emphasis on your ability to embody the basic principles of center, ground, blending, entering, and *ki* flow than on throwing your partner down. Very soon you come to the understanding that you are responsible for everything you feel, think, and do—whether in the dojo or in life.

Let's say, for example, that you are at the dojo, and because you're unable to properly execute a technique, you become frustrated and angry. A common reaction may be to complain that your training partner is too big, or you accuse them of intentionally trying to give you a hard time, or you may even try to angrily force them down. In some way or another, the tendency may be to make the situation or someone outside yourself wrong. But in reminding yourself that "the only opponent is within" and that "aikido is not for correcting others; it is for correcting your own mind," you instead face and work with your feelings of frustration and aggression. You do this first by acknowledging your aggression. Then you center yourself, move your center to the point of conflict, blend with the energy of the conflict, and finally lead this energy toward a peaceful reconciliation. This can be an internal process of working with your inner conflict, or an external process of dealing with a threat from the environment. This creates a win-win situation (in-

---

[3] Ibid, p. 177.

stead of the usual win-lose scenario), because there is no "wrong" party. When you think of the current world situation and the possibility of nuclear disaster, a win-win solution is really the only course that is sane or even applicable.

Secondly, through the different strikes, grabs, and kicks that we are exposed to in aikido, we have the opportunity to experience how we respond in confrontative situations. We can see if our reaction is to lock horns and fight back, to avoid and run away from the confrontation, or to play dumb and take no responsibility whatsoever for what is occurring.

We can also begin to see how these attacks and our responses are metaphors for situations in our daily life. By practicing the basic principles of aikido, in and out of the dojo, it is entirely possible to learn to deal with an abusive verbal attack in the same way we deal with someone punching us in the face. Aikido is a way of learning to responsibly resolve conflict without violating or dominating others, and thus our practice begins to affect our daily life.

Thirdly, aikido offers us a way of experiencing and releasing our violence in a ritualized way. In the role of *uke*, there is permission to manifest our aggression in various attacks. The role of *nage* gives permission to throw your partner, pin them to the ground, or hold them neutralized in a joint-lock. The release of this aggression, however, is acted out in the context of cooperation. In a partnership of ritualized violence, the roles of *uke* and *nage* become important instruments in teaching us how to cooperatively shape ourselves while releasing our aggression. There is, in other words, an understanding that, regardless of how intense it becomes, the exchange between *uke* and *nage* will not result in a fight. Whenever a partner wants to stop the action, the nonverbal cue in aikido is to tap the mat, yourself, or your partner. This appeasement cue is agreed upon and respected by all aikido practitioners. When aikidoists see or hear this tap, they will immediately stop what they are doing.

Studies in group psychology have long shown that the urge toward cooperation is deep-seated and is often mobilized when there is an external enemy or "other." This urge toward cooperative behavior is, ironically, one of the things that makes war possible. It is interesting to consider that perhaps our personal and global challenge lies in responding to this cooperative urge without making someone else wrong or creating an enemy. Aikido, with the dual roles of *uke* and *nage*, offers the opportunity to explore our aggressive side while retaining the context of cooperating. From one point of view, aikido can be seen as a way for two people to cooperate with each other in the safe exploration of their aggression.

The other day, when someone defined peace as a time without conflict, some faraway paradise momentarily seemed to pass before his eyes. He hinted at a place where, once and for all, we would all settle onto forty acres of tension-free bliss, a time when conflict would have finally run its course, and after having come to our senses, we would live peacefully ever after. Unfortunately, there is nothing in nature or history to indicate that anything at all is so static and unchanging. Our hopes for a new order are important, but our actions are what will bring the vision into our neighborhood. Our aggressiveness is as much a part of our nature as is peace. Aggressiveness simply is, and it can be worked with in our bodies and minds. Peace, in much the same way, is not some final destination, but a process that we need to work with every day, every moment, in all aspects of our lives.

Aikido is a form that works with the transformation of aggression and the cultivation of harmony. What about introducing aikido in the schools around the third grade? This is the age we begin to teach aikido to children, and it seems to satisfy a deep hunger in them. They learn a number of valuable skills, like rolling and falling, mind/body harmony, and grace in movement. They are also able to make strong, but safe physical contact, to learn alternatives to fighting, and to earn their right to practice the art of self-defense.

Conclusion

To live in a human body is a rare gift. Through this situation, we experience our lives. Our bodies also carry the potential for self-knowledge, self-healing, love, and compassion. By reawakening the perceptive skills of feeling, sensing, and intuiting, we can allow the wisdom of the body to emerge, to guide and inform us.

This is both a simple and challenging task. Simple, because this wisdom is our natural birthright, not requiring any equipment other than what we already have: our bodies, energy, and awareness. At the same time, it is challenging, because the entire structure of our society runs counter to this way of life, a fact that should neither discourage us, nor turn us into hysterical revolutionaries. By working sincerely and directly with our present situation, we can begin to live in our bodies, thereby affecting our own lives, as well as the lives of others.

My hope is that this book confirms what you already know: you can trust what you feel and sense. You can allow these perceptions to enrich your life. I also ask that you listen to the ideas in this book with your heart, that you practice the exercises sincerely, and that you find a teacher who can take you further along this path. If these things happen, my intention toward you, the reader, will have been fulfilled.

Richard Heckler, a fourth degree black belt in aikido, holds a Ph.D. in psychology. He is a founding member of the Lomi School and Tamalpais Aikido Dojo in northern California. A pioneer in the theraputic use of aikido, bodywork and meditative disciplines, he has worked with emotionally disturbed children, inner-city gangs, professional athletes, the Army Special Forces, and the Navy S.E.A.L.S. He is the author of two previous books, *Aikido and the New Warrior* and *In Search of the Warrior Spirit*.